T0342444

IN THE TIME OF EBOLA

IN THE TIME OF EBOLA

Youth, Family, and Emergency in Sierra Leone

Jonah Lipton

CORNELL UNIVERSITY PRESS   **ITHACA AND LONDON**

First published 2024 by Cornell University Press

Library of Congress Cataloging-in-Publication Data

Names: Lipton, Jonah, 1988– author.
Title: In the time of Ebola : youth, family, and emergency in Sierra Leone / Jonah Lipton.
Description: Ithaca [New York] : Cornell University Press, 2024. | Includes bibliographical references and index.
Identifiers: LCCN 2024004828 (print) | LCCN 2024004829 (ebook) | ISBN 9781501778094 (hardcover) | ISBN 9781501778100 (paperback) | ISBN 9781501778117 (epub) | ISBN 9781501778124 (pdf)
Subjects: LCSH: Ebola virus disease—Social aspects—Sierra Leone. | Epidemics—Social aspects—Sierra Leone—History—21st century. | Epidemics—Economic aspects—Sierra Leone—History—21st century. | Epidemics—Africa, West—History—21st century.
Classification: LCC RC140.5 .L57 2024 (print) | LCC RC140.5 (ebook) | DDC 616.9/18009664—dc23/eng/20240408
LC record available at https://lccn.loc.gov/2024004828
LC ebook record available at https://lccn.loc.gov/2024004829

In memory of James Conteh, Andrew Lebby, and Peter Lipton

Contents

Acknowledgments

I am grateful to all of those at the London School of Economics, past and present, who have supported this book throughout the years. Thank you Deborah James and Matthew Engelke for your long-term guidance since my time in the Department of Anthropology. I am thankful for the support of my colleagues at the Firoz Lalji Institute for Africa and the Centre for Public Authority and International Development, in particular Tim Allen, Martha Geiger, and Melissa Parker.

I am greatly appreciative to all of those, more than can be mentioned here, who have read my work and supported this research from its inception until its finished form. I would particularly like to mention Adia Benton, Thomas Brooks, Charlotte Bruckermann, Michael Edwards, Harri Englund, Ilana Gershon, Hyman Gross, Aisha Ibrahim, Marloes Janson, Melissa Lane, Nick Long, Fabio Mattioli, Friederike Mieth, the anonymous reviewers at the *Journal of the Royal Anthropological Institute* and *American Ethnologist*, and the two reviewers of this manuscript.

I have benefited from the comments and feedback from audiences at the London School of Economics, Cambridge University, St. Peter's College Oxford, the University of Melbourne, La Trobe University, Njala University, the Max Planck Institute for Social Anthropology, the University of Bath, the London School of Hygiene and Tropical Medicine, and several conferences.

I am indebted to my friends in Freetown, who generously accepted me into their lives and guided me through my fieldwork with care and humor. They have not only shaped the contents of this book but have also taught me lessons that have shaped my life.

I am so grateful for the love of my friends and family. Diana Lipton, Jacob Lipton, and my partner, Eda Seyhan, have engaged deeply with me in this work and supported and facilitated it in innumerable other ways. Thank you Hatice, Nail, and Jale for hosting me in Naarm (Melbourne), where much of this book was written.

The writing of and research for this book were supported by the UK Economic and Social Research Council, which funds the Centre for Public Authority and International Development research grants ES/P008038/1 and ES/W00786X/1. Earlier research funding came from the Horowitz Foundation for Social Policy, a Malinowski Memorial Grant, a Halperin Memorial Fund Pre-Doctoral

Travel Fellowship, a Rosemary and Raymond Firth Scholarship, and an Alfred Gell Memorial Studentship.

Parts of this book have been published in different forms, and I appreciate the permission given to reuse this work in its new form. A different version of chapter 5 was published with the title "'Black' and 'White' Death: Burials in a Time of Ebola in Freetown, Sierra Leone" in the *Journal of the Royal Anthropological Institute* 23, no. 4 (2017): 801–19. Some of the ethnographic material presented in chapter 4 appears in a chapter titled "Taking Life 'Off Hold': Pregnancy and Family Formation during the Ebola Crisis in Freetown, Sierra Leone" in the book *Pregnant in the Time of Ebola: Women and Their Children in the 2013–2015 West African Epidemic*, edited by David A. Schwartz, Julienne Ngoundoung Anoko, and Sharon A. Abramowitz (Cham, Switzerland: Springer Nature, 2019).

Names have been changed to protect people's identity.

Kamara Family

Foday (young taxi driver and musician)
Molay (Foday's grandfather)
Umaru (a comedian and Foday's elder cousin)
Sam (Foday's younger cousin)
Alhassan (a taxi driver and Foday's elder brother)

Bangura Family

James (young cook)
Leah (a cook and James's stepmother)
Marie (Leah's younger sister)
Kadiatu (Leah's niece)
Aisha (a market trader and James's partner)
Zainab (young hotel receptionist)

Cole Family

Brima (police officer)
Sally (Brima's wife)
Andrew (a retired police officer and Brima's uncle)
Fatu (a shopkeeper and Brima's aunt)

Other Characters

Human Right (motorbike taxi driver)
Balloon Burst (young apprentice)
Councilor (Sierra Leone Commercial Bike Riders Union [BRU] official)

Peter (BRU Union officer, university student, and bike rider in Ebola burial team)

Alimamy (bike rider in Ebola burial team)

INTRODUCTION

This is a book about the 2014–2016 West African Ebola epidemic. However, it is an unusual account of a major global health crisis. Rather than beginning with the outbreak of a novel virus and then telling the story of the devastation it caused and the responses of various government officials, public health professionals, and humanitarian organizations, this story centers on the residents of an ordinary neighborhood in a city that became unexpectedly swept up in the emergency. The central protagonists are young men and women and their families, neighbors, and friends with whom I lived for two years in Freetown, Sierra Leone's capital city. Many aspects of day-to-day life are covered here, such as routines around the home, work, and romantic and familial relationships as well as sickness and death. I also include an account of my own experience of being an anthropologist doing fieldwork during an unexpected emergency. In other words, the stories here are in several respects ordinary stories that take place in an extraordinary time and immediately before and after.

This orientation is valuable in several ways. First, it aims to bridge the alarming disconnect between the ways that emergencies such as Ebola are talked about and conceptualized in academic, public, and indeed private forums and most people's lived experiences of them. Emergencies tend to be described as dramatic and shocking events that represent disturbing aberrations from normality. Yet, for many people normal times contain challenges that actually exceed those faced during emergencies, not least because there is no clear end in sight. While sickness, loss, and other destabilizing forces are widespread during emergencies, many people's experiences are better characterized by more prosaic and repetitive patterns of social activity and care. In some cases, including for many young people in Sierra Leone during the Ebola epidemic, emergencies present greater social clarity and possibility than is normally available. Yet, we seem to lack the discourse and perhaps the inclination to bring the full spectrum of ordinary experiences of emergency into serious dialogue with extraordinary framings that continue to dominate not only the ways we narrate and think about emergencies but also how official responses are set up.

Second and connected to this point, this book helps us better understand how health emergencies are structured by and experienced in relation to a much wider and subtler set of forces and concerns than public health and biomedicine. Here I am particularly interested in the time of emergency as a principally social, political, and economic time that is mutually constituted between a wide range of actors in rather nonstraightforward ways. Dominant academic and critical models for the broader context of emergency tend to emphasize its vertical dimensions: how emergencies further the projects of domination by economic and political elites and how the marginalized suffer and fight back. These are critical dynamics that cannot be overlooked. What is missing, however, are the social, relational, and intimate spheres—particularly those of family and home—that are connected to but not contained within the more vertical and macro models. Activity and agency in these spheres tend to be more coded and nonlinear than at the macro level and, perhaps due to difficulties of access in many research methodologies, go widely unacknowledged and underappreciated despite being definitive of most people's day-to-day experiences of emergencies and their aftermath.

This book is partly intended for scholars and students of anthropology, African studies, and related disciplines by extending and rethinking our empirical and theoretical understandings of crisis, youth, and family life in Africa in part through interrogating how Ebola and emergencies more generally are experienced and shaped by people who are already in "crisis" of one sort or another. In doing so, the book brings together insights from various traditions of anthropology, including social, economic, medical, and cultural. At the same time, the book is intended for a broader audience without great familiarity with these fields who are interested in knowing what the 2014–2016 West African Ebola epidemic looked like on the ground and contains useful lessons for practitioners and policy makers on the value of long-standing anthropological methods and insights for building better responses to epidemics and other emergencies. Yet, ultimately this book aims to reveal how ordinary people's responses to a health emergency point us to deeper crises that demand radical solutions.

It was midafternoon, and I was slouching on the side of Foday's bed. Foday was a part-time taxi driver and an aspiring recording artist in his early twenties. He was hosting me in his small home during my long-term fieldwork in Freetown, Sierra Leone's bustling capital city. We were scrolling through new messages on one of his WhatsApp groups, named "One Love" and composed mostly of friends and family from the neighborhood. Amid the regular greetings and jokes on the thread were some alarming photographs of a man lying on the ground, blood pouring out of his orifices. An accompanying message reported a new deadly virus discovered across the Guinea border. Foday, with slight comic exaggeration, exclaimed, "Why always Africa?!" After a short back-and-forth, we concluded that it was most likely fake news designed to go viral, and Foday continued scrolling.

It was not fake news. A few months later in August 2014, the World Health Organization labeled the West African Ebola outbreak a public health emergency of international concern. It would be the largest outbreak of the Ebola virus disease in recorded history. Ebola is a zoonotic disease, transmitted from wild animals to humans. Ebola primarily spreads through human populations by contact with the bodily fluids of an infected person who is symptomatic with or has succumbed to the disease. Symptoms include fever, headache, vomiting, and diarrhea as well as internal and external bleeding. Patients can become severely dehydrated, and their immune systems can be highly compromised. By the time of the West African outbreak, survival rates of those infected with Ebola was less than 50 percent, a figure improved with good rehydration treatment. Despite earlier outbreaks on the continent that were considerably smaller, there was no available vaccine in 2014. This was the result of both limited opportunities to conduct trials and the business models of private pharmaceutical companies, which were set up to capitalize on an eventual major outbreak when major public funding for vaccine development would be unlocked.[1]

Sierra Leone, which was at the epicenter of the outbreak along with Guinea and Liberia, declared a national state of emergency. A humanitarian and public health intervention consisting of scores of international state and nongovernmental bodies landed in Freetown, costing more than $3.5 billion in total.[2] A few Ebola cases were reported in our neighborhood in Freetown, leading to the quarantining of several homes, but the virus did not spread as it did elsewhere in the country. Ultimately, the World Health Organization recorded close to four thousand deaths from ten thousand Ebola cases in 2014–2016 in Sierra Leone, a country with an estimated population of seven million.

Millions were affected by the epidemic and the global response to it in other ways. Ebola caused only 14 percent of deaths in the country at the time (malaria, which is absolutely routine in much of Africa, caused 27%).[3] For Foday and other residents of the neighborhood, the term "Ebola"—meaning not just the epidemic but all that the emergency came to signify—became an unavoidable part of everyday life. Quarantines and curfews were commonplace. Life-course rituals, particularly funerals, were subject to novel regulations and protocols. Work and education were suspended for many, while others gained formal employment for the first time in the official Ebola response. The bylaws, material flows, and new bureaucratic structures of the state of emergency would last for forty-two days after the last confirmed Ebola case, double the incubation period of the virus, in a moving horizon that was eventually reached after just over two years.

When I began this research project, I did not anticipate that I would eventually write a book about a global health emergency. I had not even heard of the Ebola virus and knew very little about epidemiology. However, the fact that I was in the unusual position to research a major emergency in Africa from the revealing vantage point of an ordinary urban community caught up in it was not completely coincidental. As I discovered, the anthropological methodologies in which I had been trained contained both the capacity for flexibility and the high degree of social embeddedness, or grounding, that allowed the research project to orient toward a turn of events that nobody expected.

During emergencies there is often demand for rapid data collection and policy-oriented research, while more open-ended methodologies are regularly sidelined. The reasons for this bias are somewhat understandable. Policy makers and agencies are tasked with making quick decisions. At the same time, during emergencies there can be greater practical and ethical challenges in longer-term and socially embedded research methodologies. The problem, however, is that rapid and policy-oriented research tends to project narrow visions of society that focus on single predetermined issues (such as a dangerous disease) and selective groups of people (the influence of international actors is often sidelined in African-based research). Research subjects are given little agency in shaping the direction or emphasis of the study, and they rarely tell us much about deeper problems that underlie the emergency in question. How "emergency" has been framed and whose interests such framings serve are rarely critically examined. To really speak to these issues requires the freedom of a looser and more open-ended approach in which the researcher is not materially dependent on any intervening agency and has developed meaningful personal relationships in the research site. This book is in part a case for the enduring usefulness of established anthropological and ethnographic methods in understanding contemporary emergencies.[4]

The central method that I used in the research for this book is known as "participant observation," developed by social and cultural anthropologists during the first half of the twentieth century. The method has been tweaked and refined over the past century, but the basics remain the same. Anthropologists spend an extended period of time, normally between one and two years, living with a group of people, learning the local language(s) and ways of living, and building a network of relationships along the way. These people tend to become the anthropologists' primary interlocutors, or research subjects. Anthropologists record what their research subjects tell them about their lives and worlds while also noting what they directly observe from participating alongside them. These findings are written in the anthropologists' field notes, which are normally structured like a diary with daily entries.

I spent two years in total doing fieldwork in Freetown over a seven-year period, with the bulk of the research taking place between 2013 and 2015. My primary field site was in the Congo Town neighborhood, home to roughly twenty thousand residents, where I lived throughout the research. Because the project was grounded as much as possible in the lived realities of those around me, its focus shifted over time. This is a common experience for anthropologists, although it does not normally happen in quite such a dramatic way as I experienced. My research project began as a study of young men in Freetown's informal economy, with a focus on taxi drivers. In the aftermath of the Sierra Leone Civil War, many youths, including former rebel soldiers, migrated to cities in search of opportunity. Many found themselves working as drivers. I started out living in Foday's small two-room home in the Congo Town neighborhood of Freetown along with two of his cousins. I was introduced to Foday by my brother, Jacob, who became close with his family when he was living in Freetown some years earlier while working in Sierra Leone's Ministry of Foreign Affairs. Foday was a young taxi driver and was a useful connection for starting my fieldwork. Over time I developed personal relationships with many people in and beyond Foday's network of family and friends, most of whom were based in or connected to the neighborhood where we lived. I am still regularly in touch with many of these people today.

I learned a lot about the taxi driving business in Freetown by interviewing and hanging out with drivers on the streets, some of which features in this book. But as time went on, this felt less significant and interesting to me than what I was seeing and participating in and around Foday's home. I regularly shared food and company with our neighbors, who invited me to family events such as baby-naming ceremonies, weddings, and funerals. I assisted with household tasks, from buying and preparing food to helping children with their schoolwork. I would shoot the breeze with aunts and uncles on their verandas, looping into the latest neighborhood gossip, and pass the time with young guys at hang-out spots known as "long-bench," where endless debates were held about the about the relative superiority of the footballers Messi and Ronaldo and other similarly inconclusive topics. My days became filled with the "full-time job" of keeping up with the demands and unpredictable rhythms of a thick web of neighborly relationships. Some days were slow and boring, and other days were highly dramatic and fraught.

The Ebola outbreak came nine months into my longest stint of fieldwork. This did not mean that I had to give up what I had been doing and start again from scratch, although I certainly encountered obstacles along the way and needed to make compromises in order to minimize risks. The gradual evolution of my research project prior to the epidemic allowed me to study it in a unique way. The emergency shone a revealing spotlight on many of the issues and social dynamics that I had already been observing. My social network in Freetown, particularly in the Congo Town neighborhood, became the locus for examining the emergency's meaning and impact for ordinary residents as well as the ways that they responded to and shaped it in their own terms. Having developed a lived understanding of day-to-day life in the community prior to the outbreak, I was able to assess its real significance in ways that beginning an Ebola-focused study during the epidemic would not allow for.

Emergency and "Crisis"

Sometimes Freetown felt to me like a forgotten or neglected city, a notion that its residents would often complain about. The city has deep cosmopolitan roots, but these are buried beneath crumbling infrastructure, crowded residential areas, and overstretched health systems. Freetown was founded by Black settlers from London in the late eighteenth century as a refuge for former slaves. Not long after it was ceded to the British Empire, becoming the capital of British West Africa. With a large natural harbor and port, Freetown attracted migrants and merchants from inland and overseas. Sierra Leone gained independence in 1961 but by the 1980s was marred by economic decline and political collapse, in part the result of international neoliberal and arguably neocolonial demands for extractive economic arrangements based around mining and the reduction of state spending and capacity. Global economic and political structures continue to ensure that only a meager percentage of Sierra Leone's considerable wealth in natural resources benefits the country's ordinary citizens.

Before Ebola, the last time Sierra Leone was in the global spotlight for a sustained period was during its decade-long civil war at the end of the twentieth century. This began as a youth uprising in response to exploitative local agrarian economies and a weak and corrupt national political system. The war was fueled by international sanctions and economic collapse and ended with a high-profile liberal peace-building intervention out of Freetown. Outright violence might now be mostly suppressed, but daily struggle, vast economic inequality, and an underresourced and exploitative state apparatus persist. Communities suffer from flooding, fire, and other environmental disasters on an almost

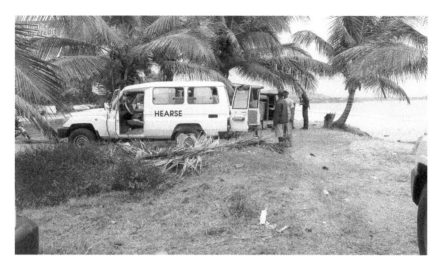

FIGURE 1. The makeshift base of an Ebola burial team.

annual basis. Most young people whom I know dream of overseas migration, seeing it as practically the only route for long-term social mobility and material security for their families. At the same time, they pursue piecemeal, nonlinear journeys of coming of age in town, negotiating precarious work and education, ambiguous and yet caring familial and domestic relationships, and the often messy business of intimate partnerships and raising children.

During the 2014–2016 Ebola epidemic, the global spotlight shone on Sierra Leone once more. International agencies such as the World Health Organization, the United Nations, the UK Ministry of Defense, and the US-based Centers for Disease Control and Prevention set up camp in hotels, ministries, and the vacated offices of the Special Court for Sierra Leone, where twenty-three former rebel soldiers were tried for international war crimes between 2002 and 2013, as well as in more makeshift settings around town (see figure 1). The rarity of Ebola, combined with its disturbing and often deadly symptoms, dominated the way the epidemic was covered by the media and how the global response was set up. The few cases that did reach North America and Europe sparked considerable panic, despite Ebola's relatively low risk of contagion as a nonairborne virus. The global response to the epidemic, which was initially criticized for being slow off the mark, ultimately entailed the mass mobilization of military, health, and humanitarian agencies with a highly securitized agenda.

Ironically, many of the conditions that rendered the Ebola emergency "extraordinary" were routinely familiar for residents of the countries at its epicenter (and for many people across the globe today): inadequate public health care, the overcrowding of cities, and the rapidly growing levels of exploitation and destruction of nature. In the rural borderland region of Libera, Sierra Leone, and Guinea, where the 2014 Ebola outbreak began, there are plenty of recent and historical reasons to mistrust the state and other bureaucratic and foreign entities, not least of which was the Atlantic slave trade that ravaged the region and casts a long shadow. And there are well-developed social systems to operate outside of or in negotiation with external control.[5] On top of this, the state and international measures employed during the emergency were remarkably old-fashioned, seemingly unbeknownst to most of the actors involved. The lockdowns, quarantines, community mapping, and centralized management of burials were strikingly reminiscent of British colonial approaches to epidemic management, including during the great influenza epidemic that hit the region a century earlier.[6]

After the state of emergency was declared in August 2014, with the epidemic rolling on for several years, the term "Ebola" took on a wide range of meanings in Freetown. For example, when there was a death in the neighborhood and the body was buried by official burial teams according to the state of emergency protocols, the deceased was often described as an Ebola victim even if it was medically determined that the person had died from another cause. Although the majority of those who died in the country between 2014 and 2016 did so from routine, if preventable, causes, being buried as if they had Ebola—intended as a safety precaution—rendered them Ebola victims in many people's eyes. There was a similar pattern for sickness. During a phone conversation with Alhassan (Foday's older brother), who was convinced that he had a routine case of malaria and was concerned about being misdiagnosed as being positive for Ebola, he expressed it to me like this: "Ebola is the only illness in Sierra Leone right now."

But the meaning of the term "Ebola" went beyond even death and illness. When people materially benefited from Ebola aid packages or employment in the official response, as a number of people in the neighborhood did, they were described as "eating Ebola money." Equally, when young people complained about Ebola, they were often referring to loss of livelihood, experiencing boredom, and lack of adequate health care or, in a more amorphous way, lack of opportunity. On one level, "Ebola" referred to a wide array of aspects of life and death in the time of Ebola, many of them byproducts of an epidemiologically focused intervention and state of emergency. On another level, "Ebola" was a new way of talking about and responding to shortcomings that are an ordinary and familiar part of life in Sierra Leone. The range of interpretations and meanings given to the term "Ebola" by those living in its proximity point to something more than the singular public health crisis that Ebola was internationally understood to be.

I argue that the Ebola emergency in Sierra Leone was really the coming to-gether of two different forms of crisis: one an unusual and temporary epidemic, the other familiar and ongoing "crisis."[7] The former crisis is the disruptive epidemic that dominated international attention. Its contours were determined by a biomedical metric of active Ebola cases in human populations, an easily definable and quantifiable standard, although there were challenges in testing and reporting cases. The boundaries of the Ebola epidemic were laid out by agencies such as the World Health Organization and, in turn, by national authorities. In Sierra Leone, the bylaws and political structures of the state of emergency were to be lifted forty-two days after the last detected case of Ebola, which is double the twenty-one-day incubation period of the virus. While this was a rolling horizon that was continually pushed back when new cases were identified—and there was quite a lot of speculation on the ground that the beneficiaries of the state of emergency were fudging the numbers so that it was prolonged—it was nonetheless definitionally and ultimately temporary. This version of Ebola as an epidemic fits the classic mold of crisis as an exceptional period of disorder or rupture. The epidemic's temporariness and medical connotations are captured in the ancient Greek term *krisis*, meaning "the turning point in a disease." The "emergent" in emergency speaks to Ebola's imminent and passing qualities.[8]

In contrast to Ebola as an epidemic that in a certain respect "came out of no-where," and would ultimately be declared over, the term "Ebola," as my interlocutors in Freetown rendered it, was meaningful in relation to ongoing social, economic, and political processes. The term signified the novelties of life (and death) during the emergency while also being mobilized as a new way of talking about and responding to "old normal" problems. This version of Ebola maps onto contemporary critical readings of crisis as the norm rather than the exception.[9] Here "crisis" is multifaceted, connected to the extending and deepening of capitalism in the post–Cold War era through which arrangements of work and care are restructured while community and state-based safety nets become overstretched or torn apart. Material inequalities and disparities have grown, while openings for social mobility have shrunk. Climate catastrophe looms, while political and economic institutions built around capitalist principles of competition and growth continually prove ill-equipped to reverse it. "Crisis" as a subjective experience in contemporary renderings has enduring, slow-burning qualities in which people are forced to "wait" or become "stuck."[10] In Africa, youths are the posterchildren of "crisis." In what is often referred to as the "crisis of youth," "lost generations" of young people find themselves without the material and symbolic resources required to achieve "social adulthood." In one interpretation, African youths confront the immobility of "waithood," while in another they navigate the constantly shifting terrain of "crisis as context."[11]

By exploring young people's lives during the Ebola emergency in Sierra Leone, this book examines what happens when a temporary epidemic and ongoing "crisis" come together. I highlight the multifaceted outcomes of this interaction for ordinary people whose lives became entangled within their meeting. While the international agencies' priorities were the short-term management of the epidemic, ordinary people tended to have longer-term priorities that went beyond the containment of the outbreak. The emergency had, of course, narrowing and restrictive elements to it but, paradoxically, also presented people with unusual clarity on many of the ambiguities and inequities of normal life. The novel bureaucracies of the official Ebola response were not yet fully tainted with the patterns of exclusion that the marginalized are accustomed to, while collective attention across many strata of society was unusually aligned toward a pressing and unfolding problem. This had ramifications that went well beyond the containment of an unusual disease not only in political and economic shifts within a state of emergency but also in a particularly profound way to the intimate social realities of ordinary people. For young people such as Foday who had struggled to fulfill inherited expectations to start families, find jobs, and progress through the life course in a dignified way, the Ebola emergency represented one of a multitude of obstacles and unusual pathways for living an "ordinary life" in a challenging place and time.

Youth in Africa: A Return to the Family

When people ask me what it is like to live in Freetown, I normally try to convey something of the struggle and hardship that ordinary people face there, combined with the nurturing and supportive bonds of community, friendship, and family that I have witnessed and experienced. Well before the Ebola emergency, I was struck by the ambiguities of life in and around the homes that I stayed in and frequented.[12] Family and domestic spaces were havens of care and generosity, but they were also sites of competition and danger. For the young people I was closest to, money, food, things, and work typically came to them through networks of family, friends, and neighbors. But in receiving gifts and opportunities, they risked becoming overly indebted. Becoming respected adults demanded that they become to some degree independent, setting up their own homes and supporting others "beneath" them rather than staying at home and being overly dependent on those "above" them.

To understand any emergency requires understanding the conditions of life that surround it. In this account, young people provide a through line that connects life before, during, and after Ebola. The protagonists in this book were in their late teens or their twenties and thirties during the time of my fieldwork. This suited my research process as a relatively young person myself. It made social sense for me to integrate into an age set in the neighborhood, and some of the deepest friendships I formed were with people of a similar age. This demographic also represents a large swath of Freetown's population, with young people continuing to migrate to the capital city in search of opportunity and with life-expectancy being only fifty-five years.

I discovered that youths occupy unusually helpful subject positions to shed light on questions about the social dynamics of an emergency in Africa. African youths are widely understood by anthropologists and other social scientists as being stuck in a "crisis of social reproduction," unable to achieve "social adult-hood."[13] During the Ebola emergency young people played critical and high-profile roles in the official as well as unofficial responses. I argue that the home and the family are central to both of these stories of crisis in ways that have been widely overlooked. In Freetown, the domestic spheres were where Ebola transmission and dynamics of containment played out most prominently. The significance of these spaces during the epidemic was magnified by their long-standing place as the front line in young people's struggles to come of age in socially respectable ways.

The difficulties that youths in Africa face in achieving social adulthood have become a well-documented phenomenon in recent decades. The United Nations labels Africa the "world's youngest continent," with 60 percent of the population under the age of twenty-five.[14] In European colonial discourse, Africa and its inhabitants were imagined as "childlike" and "undeveloped," representations that supported coercive colonization. Africa's contemporary crisis of youth is widely connected to the legacy of structural adjustment reforms during the 1980s and 1990s, spearheaded by the International Monetary Fund and the World Bank, during which drastic cuts were made to state budgets and capacities across the Global South in a bid to shore up free market economic growth. In most cases the results were devastating, with economic activity becoming increasingly extractive rather than trickling down to ordinary people, as neoliberalism's advocates promised. At the same time, anticorruption initiatives actively targeted the patrimonial networks through which resources are informally distributed from "big men" to clients, many of them poor youths. In Sierra Leone, this paved the way for the civil war during the 1990s and early 2000s as disenfranchised youths formed rebel groups, allowing them to live outside of and in opposition to the neglectful and oppressive institutions of the state and rural society.[15]

Partly as a result of a number of high-profile youth-led armed uprisings and protest movements from the 1990s to the present across the continent, there has been a propensity in international popular culture, journalism, and scholarship to frame African youths, particularly males, as violent actors. Even sympathetic accounts that usefully highlight how violence is not an innate quality of African youth cultures but instead is a consequence of political and economic marginalization still risk inadvertently reproducing this basic framing. In scholarship, young men such as street hustlers and vigilantes are often studied in public male-dominated contexts and spaces.

Domestic spaces of the home and family are strikingly underrepresented in studies of contemporary male youth (with some notable recent exceptions) even though these spaces are of central significance in many aspects of young people's lives. This omission is all the more striking given that earlier anthropological work on youth in Africa focused almost entirely on the sphere of family (or "kinship" as it was termed). Kinship was the defining political and economic institution in pastoral and agrarian societies, and even research in urban settings emphasized its primacy.[16] The apparent assumption that family and kinship are no longer significant spheres for those incorporated into state and global political and economic structures misses the lived reality of young people in cities such as Freetown who are not simply connected to domestic and familial networks but are utterly reliant on them. While the crisis of youth is a story about a generation cutting loose and getting lost, it is also a story about coming home if indeed they left in the first place.

On a basic level, unemployed and irregularly employed young men in Freetown tend to spend a lot of time at home. Formal employment is much less available now in the aftermath of shrinking industrial production in the city and trade through the port. As noted above, the thick relationships that Freetown youths form with family, friends, and neighbors are not only important for managing the spaces of home and daily sustenance—whether this involves the sharing of food or other acts of care and mutual support—but are also central to business opportunities and the management of informal work. On one side of the coin, familial, domestic, and neighborly relationships represent possibility for young people in Freetown, encapsulated by the Krio term *sababu*, which translates as "beneficial relationship" and "luck." On the other side, such relationships can easily lead to indebtedness, infantilization, and ultimately the form of stuckedness that many youths desire to escape.[17] The paradox that many young people find themselves in might be best expressed this way: You need family to make it in business, and you need business to make it in family.

The significance of home and family for young people in Freetown did not diminish during the Ebola emergency. Rather, their stakes became even higher. Ebola was sometimes described as a "family disease" in Sierra Leone, as the virus commonly spread between intimate relations, typically through acts of care for the sick and dead (in preparing corpses for burial). Such activities are normally performed by family and others close by rather than health care professionals. Family gatherings, particularly burials, risked becoming so-called superspreader events, as there were often strong obligations for even distantly located relatives to attend. Ebola was described as being cruel in the ways that it punished acts of care and coming close in times of crisis.

During the state of emergency, public authorities from the state, nongovernmental organizations (NGOs), and international agencies scrutinized and regulated many aspects of domestic and family life. New ways of performing safe burials were devised under the auspices of official burial teams, composed mostly of young men employed and managed by the state and NGOs. Neighborhoods and homes were routinely monitored by authorities during lockdowns, quarantines, and curfews. Health services could be contacted by ordinary people from home through the 117 emergency service, which was nonexistent before Ebola.

Critical accounts and sympathetic campaigns have highlighted the difficult dimensions of both the epidemic itself and the international and local responses to it. Some reports point to Ebola victims becoming stigmatized in communities after they had recovered (this is not something that I came across firsthand).[18] Others highlight the intrusive characteristics of the official Ebola response, which placed severe limitations on people's lives and in some cases was an obstacle to grassroots responses and initiatives.[19] Many of these negative features of epidemiological responses were not novel to Ebola but are connected to deeply grooved historical patterns. Critical studies repeatedly point to the ways that epidemics trace existing social inequalities and fault lines, such as around sexuality, race, generation, and class.[20] Systems of public and global health create or extend inequalities through measures that disproportionally disadvantage some groups over others. That so many historical mistakes were repeated during the COVID-19 pandemic is a sober reminder of what work remains to be done.

In Freetown, some of the core social dynamics around Ebola were remarkably consistent with those that preceded it. The ambiguities of home during Ebola, as a space of both refuge and danger, were reminiscent of similar dynamics for youths beforehand. The overlaps were brought home to me early on in the stage of the emergency when the virus had still not spread into Freetown. A girl living next door to the family compound I was staying in suffered an attack of witchcraft, revealed by three marks that appeared on her back. In the weeks and months that followed, my neighbors hired a witchdoctor who led dramatic nightlong sessions to lure the invisible witches and protect the residents. There was a suspicion that one of the neighbors was living a double life as a witch, although there was no final agreement about who this was. This notion of witchcraft as an invisible expression of ill will or jealousy from those close by, the "enemy within," is a common trope in Africa and its diaspora.[21] It turned out that this established framework and the underlying social reality it referenced were quite applicable to Ebola, which similarly traveled through networks of intimacy. Both witchcraft and Ebola revealed vulnerabilities of intimacy that were already there, finding expression in many aspects of young people's day-to-day lives. Surviving "Ebola" was a matter of not only avoiding contact with the virus but also realigning intimate and familial relationships in ways that lasted well beyond the epidemic. Acts of social realignment tied into a wider reconfiguring of hierarchy and established protocols during the state of emergency, undergirded by new bylaws, public authority structures, and material flows.

In Freetown, the form that these intimate realignments took was not the radical reimaginings or rejections of traditional ways of doing that might be expected by youths in a global emergency. Rather, they were strikingly traditional and ordinary in their orientation, albeit creative and adaptive.[22] In Freetown, young people found renewed potency and possibility in life-course rituals, family formation, formal waged work, and bureaucratic workings of the state. It is no coincidence that these were all features of life that many young people valued and sought out prior to the emergency but had often found to be absent or working against them. In this book, youths provide a revealing perspective on a global health emergency, while Ebola is an illuminating case study for reexamining the crisis of youth in Africa today.

What Is Ordinary?

This book is about ordinary life in an emergency. But what does "ordinary" mean? And why is this perspective useful? Before addressing these questions, it is helpful to first consider the two most prevalent critical models for thinking about emergencies, which we can refer to as "continuity" and "break." "Continuity" sees the emergency as a sharper and more severe version of what precedes it. Proponents of such an analysis point to the ways that the emergency reenforces or extends existing social and economic inequalities, such as through narrow and rushed responses or through intentional opportunism by elites. "Break" sees the emergency as a rupture with the status quo, as a truly exceptional period of time in which routines are disturbed and hierarchies are unsettled in fundamental ways. In this model, emergencies can have lasting, transformative, and even revolutionary potential.

Both models of emergency are plausible and historically identifiable. The problem is that they are rarely articulated in ways that are compatible with one another; whereas in all likelihood both dynamics—continuity and break—are at play simultaneously. There is a great temptation for people to apply their focus selectively, ignoring the evidence that points the other way. Quantitative data over a long time frame might identify trends that genuinely support one interpretation over the other. Ethnographic research, however, which is undertaken by the researcher over a relatively short period of time and in which the collected data is highly qualitative, tends to paint a more ambiguous picture whereby both continuities and ruptures are indeterminately there and mutually contingent. Such was my own experience of fieldwork in Freetown.

To form an analysis of emergency that accounts for both continuity and break, we need to pay much more attention to the ordinary.[23] Such an undertaking has several dimensions to it. First, it means paying attention to so-called ordinary people. In the context of an epidemic, it means looking beyond those infected with the disease or who are proximate to it in other ways, to include people whose lives are less overtly impacted by the broader emergency but who ultimately do play a large role in shaping its outcome. It means understanding how people situate the emergency within a broader ecology of concerns, needs, demands, and expectations in their lives and how they go about attending to them. This necessitates casting our attention on ordinary practices and places, in particular daily acts of care, work, and maintenance in and around the home as well as the management of progression, or movement, through the life course. In practice, many people's direct experiences of epidemics and other emergencies are not characterized by the kind of dramatic upheavals that fuel media narratives—even though they too must contend with such narratives—but instead are largely made up of mundane time among those they live with. For those who do suffer loss and grief in emergencies, getting through it often depends on these core relationships.

Second, we must acknowledge that the term "ordinary" has multiple meanings. In any social setting, ordinary can index a valuation of a state that is normally, or ordinarily, there. This might be thought of as a sort of statistical average of reality. At the same time, ordinary is likely to index an ideal of how things should be rather than an assessment of how things typically are.[24] The mismatch between ordinary as a reality versus ordinary as an ideal seems to be particularly pronounced in recent periods of economic decline and political and ecological crisis, when difficulties in meeting inherited expectations and aspirations are widespread. On some level, however, such a tension between "as is" ordinary and "as if" ordinary is not peculiar to this moment but instead is foundational to ways that social groups operate and reproduce over time. The anthropological study of ritual—a long-standing preoccupation and specialty in the discipline—provides a useful model. Classic anthropological analysis, following Arnold van Gennep's work, connects ritual's efficacy for generating meaning among its participants and for the intergenerational transmission of social orders and values to the ways that ritual temporarily suspends or inverts normal rules and hierarchies. This is captured suggestively by the concept of liminality, the intermediate—betwixt and between—stage in ritual most famously described in Victor Turner's study of Ndembu coming-of-age ceremonies.[25] The key point here is that liminality in ritual is not the absence of normal social order, even though it might look wild as in the case of the Ndembu rites of passage, which happen in the forest rather than the village. Rather, liminality is the fleshing out of a coexisting, alternative, imaginary order. Turner describes liminality as "dominantly in the 'subjunctive mood' of culture, the mood of maybe, might-be, as-if, hypothesis, fantasy, conjecture, desire."[26] In ritual theory, these two social orders have been labeled "as is" and "as if," the former referring to the sincerity of everyday life and the latter to the play and imaginaries of ritual time.[27]

Third, we must question whose notion of ordinary is in play. Such interrogation is at the heart of the anthropological enterprise, and I believe it is one of the discipline's key contributions in understanding emergency today. In cases of foreign and top-down interventions, we question whether the understanding of "ordinary" in one group, normally the dominant actors, is being imposed onto others, normally the disempowered. The epistemic and material violence associated with this pattern cannot be overstated. However, this model risks masking the enduringness and porousness of such processes. In the context of over five hundred years of colonialization and foreign intervention in West Africa, people in Freetown tend to move between multiple overlapping social orders rather than inhabiting any singular social order or cultural framework. As others have noted, the colonial encounter in Africa has led to a great deal of intermixing between social orders, but stark imaginative dualisms between social orders associated with the colonizers and the colonized have persisted.[28] Much contemporary anthropological scholarship undertaken in diverse field sites is concerned with the ways that people live among multiple, interconnected, and porous social orders.[29] Emergencies are critical times when the boundaries between social orders are reconfigured. As the relationship between the social orders is in flux, their (co)existence becomes more visible, which allows a range of actors to creatively redefine their boundaries. And yet, this process often leaves the distinctions between social orders intact.[30]

During the Ebola emergency, residents of Freetown creatively navigated between social orders that go back to the Atlantic slave trade and centuries of colonialism and foreign intervention. The existence of different social orders was made unusually plain during the international intervention as two worlds, one "local" and "undeveloped" and the other "global" and "developed," which are common binaries found in global health discourse.[31] During the emergency my interlocutors would refer to these orders as "black" and "white," recalling the historic, racialized, violence engendered within them. But more coded manifestations of these orders were already found in many domains of social life in Freetown, including in and around the home, in informal work, and in relationships between young people and the state. For many young people who were already caught up in the deep ambiguities that living among multiple orders entails with their contradictory visions of what it means to be a respected adult, Ebola represented a time of unusual clarity and creative possibility. The social clarity that the emergency presented had material implications for those we were able to broker between social orders, drawing on long-standing approaches to social mobility and social reproduction in West Africa.[32] At the same time, the international intervention was understood by Freetown residents less as an alien imposition and more as dialect of their own cosmopolitan language.

Chapter Outline

The bulk of the chapters in the book center around ethnographic descriptions of events and unfolding stories in Freetown spanning a period of over seven years. In addition, each chapter develops analytically on the core themes and ideas that I have identified so far. Almost everything described in the book, excluding the historical material, involves happenings that I personally witnessed and participated in. Included are the interpretations and reflections of a variety of actors as they unfold. The central protagonists of the book are a group of young people I have gotten to know very well over the years, most of whom were resident in or otherwise connected to the Congo Town neighborhood. However, much attention and space is given to all those around them, people to whom I became in many cases just as close. This includes their parents, siblings, friends, cousins, aunts and uncles, neighbors, and colleagues. The ethnographic material presented here does not progress exclusively in linear time but instead coalesces around themes, people, and arenas, which are the focus of each individual chapter.

Chapter 1 sets the stage. I begin by describing my own sense of disconnect at the early stages of the Ebola epidemic while moving between ordinary homes in the Congo Town neighborhood to meetings with international Ebola responders at the Radisson Blu Hotel, physically proximate to one another yet, at first glance, distant in other ways. However, a closer inspection reveals that these two worlds are highly interconnected. I introduce Foday's home, where I first stayed, and tell the story of his grandfather's migration to the neighborhood before I delve into Freetown's deeper history, its unusual position as a site of extraction and return in the Atlantic slave trade as well as more recent histories of British colonialism, independence, conflict, and disease management. This history is essential to understanding why an underresourced and vulnerable state with a highly depleted medical infrastructure was yet again so susceptible to heavy-handed foreign intervention and, equally, how residents of Freetown, a poor yet historically cosmopolitan city, were equipped to shape how the emergency played out in their own terms. For Freetown's young residents, economic openings, the establishing and maintenance of families and homes, and notions of agency and dependence have long been bound up with and brokered through the global forces that course through the city.

Chapter 2 steps out onto the streets, centering on a group of motorbike taxi riders. The chapter begins with a rider known as Human Right, who experienced serious injury at the hands of police. This encapsulated the physical and legal risks that marginal workers face from a state that is both neglectful and coercive. I then turn to the Sierra Leone Commercial Bike Riders Union, which was formed around ex-rebel networks in the aftermath of the civil war in the early 2000s. The union provided "state-like" bureaucratic structures that aimed to protect workers' interests while also being criticized as exploitative in parallel ways to the state. The chapter then turns to Peter, a bike rider who was recruited in the official Ebola response and worked with an Ebola burial team that I regularly followed, which was his first taste of formal employment. The account presented in chapter 2 complicates dominant critiques of humanitarian and emergency responses, including Ebola, that emphasize how state and other bureaucratic entities opportunistically use emergencies to extend their reach and influence at the expense of ordinary people. Here, in a notably urban context, grassroots organizing before the outbreak was itself quite bureaucratic in form, and the bureaucratized emergency response was widely welcomed by young workers as a fairer version of the state, while those incorporated into it attempted to shape the official response in their own image.

Chapter 3 centers on the home, a central yet ambiguous space for young people in Freetown. During the Ebola emergency, people were forced to decide between caring for those close by and following official guidance that emphasized distancing from others. Contrary to public health messaging at the time, however, such ambiguities were far from novel; rather, Ebola represented a new manifestation of an old problem. I describe three conflicts of care among young people in the neighborhood and those they lived with, which boiled down to the ambiguities of living with two coexisting sets of expectation associated with the overlapping social orders of family and business. The fundamental irreconcilability of the two logics is a definitive factor in the current manifestation of what has been called the crisis of youth in Africa.

Chapter 4 describes two events in the neighborhood during Ebola. The first was a three-day lockdown in which a popular yet contentious distribution of food took place at the local mosque. The second was a large-scale baby-naming ceremony performed by James and Aisha, a young unmarried couple who had their first child during the state of emergency. These events serve to illustrate what I call the "extraordinary ordinary," referring to the unusual openings for prized notions of ordinary life to unfold during emergencies, particularly for those for whom crisis of one sort or another is more the norm rather than the exception. Although ongoing challenges and inequalities did not disappear and were in some cases exacerbated by the official Ebola response, young people discovered potential in a number of the features of the emergency, including the transformed state, the atmosphere of urgency, collective attention on the near future, and the unusual capacity for family rituals to be adapted.

Chapter 5 continues the theme of family ritual, in this case at the other end of the life course, recounting the untimely deaths of two women from the neighborhood. Marie was buried according to official Ebola protocol, while Rachel was buried in a hybrid "secret burial". Mourners of both faced unusual challenges in enacting what anthropologists term "good death" as they encountered sizable regulations on customary mortuary ritual. Yet, both burials, while fraught, remained meaningful. To unpack this, I examine the racial categories of white and black used by mourners to describe different types of burials during the emergency. Buried beneath the normative tensions engendered in these racial categories was a conflict between, on the one hand, the new authorities and protocols of the state of emergency and, on the other hand, established public authorities and bureaucratic channels. Navigating this disjuncture was a key characteristic of living through the emergency, which came to the fore when people were confronted with the demands of pressing social obligations.

In chapter 6, I describe how I navigated an unexpected emergency in the course of a long-term ethnographic research project and outline some of the key lessons I learned along the way for researching crisis. I highlight what I consider to be three core tenets of the anthropological method, which were key in producing this book: flexibility, personal relationships, and theory from the home. During emergencies it is common for anthropological research methods to be compromised in favor of rapid policy-oriented research. This chapter makes the case for not abandoning what anthropologists—and social scientists employing ethnographic methods—can uniquely bring to the table. My aim in chapter 6 is to usefully make this case to readers who are not anthropologists while also providing practical insights from my personal experiences for anthropologists and students faced with similar questions and conditions to those that I faced during Ebola.

MARGINALIZED COSMOPOLITANS

As an anthropologist who was in Sierra Leone during the Ebola outbreak, I was invited to participate in meetings with social scientists and other professionals involved in the international response. After the World Health Organization declared Ebola a public health emergency of international concern, Freetown became a hub for a large number of international organizations as part of a response costing more than $3.5 billion. One meeting I attended was in the garden of the Radisson Blu hotel by Lumley beach in western Freetown. It was a comfortable new hotel used by international professionals during the epidemic. At the other end of the beach is the Freetown golf club, established there by British military officials stationed in Sierra Leone a little less than a hundred years earlier. Walking into the air-conditioned lobby of the Radisson Blu, with Muzak gently floating around, I felt as if I could have been anywhere in the world.

The meetings at the Radisson Blu hotel felt a million miles from the Congo Town neighborhood where I was living, even though they are only a couple of miles apart. The construction of two worlds—one developed and global, the other undeveloped and local—is a common and deeply embedded feature of international interventions in Africa and in the so-called Global South more broadly. But when you look closely it becomes apparent that the worlds that are made to appear distinct during interventions are in fact highly interconnected. A number of my neighbors and interlocutors I knew well were low-paid workers at the Radisson Blu and other hotels nearby. Such day-to-day movement between spaces associated with each world—the mostly poor African neighborhood and the international chain hotel—was undergirded by a deeper cultural familiarity, which tends to go unacknowledged by international actors.

Foreign interventions are nothing new in Sierra Leone; in fact, they have been something of a constant for about half a millennium. Social systems in Freetown have developed in ways that are entirely intertwined with the dynamics of intervention. The challenging task of navigating between the boundaries of seemingly opposed social orders, connected to different social and cultural influences, is central to how young people come of age and how families are maintained in Freetown. Therefore, for ordinary residents of Freetown, the Ebola emergency was in many ways a new iteration of an old and ongoing problem. By the same token, the language of international intervention was far from unintelligible to ordinary people and instead was like a dialect of their own cosmopolitan language formed over the centuries. This chapter focuses on various aspects of this historical and contemporary context—including the civil war in the 1990s and early 2000s, the legacies of British colonialism and independence, and the buried yet ever-relevant history of the slave trade—that help us understand why this vulnerable state was so susceptible to heavy-handed foreign intervention and also how residents of Freetown, a poor yet historically cosmopolitan Atlantic port city were equipped to shape in their own terms how the Ebola emergency played out.

Another meeting I attended took place on the premises of the Special Court for Sierra Leone, where between 2002 and 2013 twenty-three former rebel soldiers were indicted for crimes against humanity. The court was established by the United Nations and the government of Sierra Leone, at a cost of roughly US$300 million. It is a large imposing complex, close to the downtown area. The central courthouse was built in an impressive modernist design and is surrounded by barbed-wire fences, security cameras, and lookout towers. During the outbreak, the complex was repurposed as the headquarters for the National Ebola Response Centre. The location was fitting. During and after the civil war a decade and half earlier, Sierra Leone was last in the international spotlight for a sustained period.

The meetings with international Ebola responders felt alien to me, which was strange given that I too was an international professional, though not on the payroll of an agency involved in the response. As an academic anthropologist, I had been living in my field site, in the Congo Town neighborhood of Freetown, for about nine months before Ebola hit Sierra Leone and was becoming accustomed to a different way of life. Both the Radisson Blu and the Special Court for Sierra Leone were only twenty minutes from my neighborhood, but although physically proximate, they felt to me strikingly distant. At that time I was living in a crowded family compound, subdivided into numerous households that were side by side. There were chickens running around, and open sewage trenches were located not far from where residents washed and cooked. Due to water shortages, we only had running water every other day; the rest of the time we used buckets, which we filled in advance. Electricity was temperamental, and power cuts were regular.

The meetings were, of course, in English. My daily life was in Krio, the English-based creole spoken in Freetown. The cultural formalities were different. In day-to-day life in Freetown, seniority must be acknowledged through appropriate greetings and terms. In the meetings, in line with Western professional protocol, participants would ask probing questions to strangers, with markers of seniority being more coded. The participants at the meetings were mostly White Americans and Europeans who were in Sierra Leone for the first time trying to get their head around how best to undertake a large-scale public health intervention across three countries in a very short time frame.

The dichotomy of two worlds has long been embedded in narratives and frameworks of global health and epidemiology. Since colonial times, public health in Africa has been inseparable from the imposition of Western and modern values on so-called primitive society. Illness in the colonial imagination was the product of being "uncivilized" and in cultural notions of Africans' "maladaptation" to modern life.[1] Contemporary virus narratives reproduce hierarchies of distinct worlds through exoticized and wild origin stories.[2] Think of the wet markets of Wuhan during COVID-19 or the rainforests of West Africa during Ebola. The root causes of the Ebola emergency were regularly framed in terms of "local" people's attachment to "backwards" practices and customs, such as eating bushmeat, relying on home-based care for the sick, and washing the bodies of the deceased.

In these deep-rooted frameworks of global health, the "cure" is implicitly, if not explicitly, modernity. This can come in the form of an intervention armed with the latest epidemiological technology, from the involvement of "modern" people (read: Westerners or White people), or through bureaucratic and biomedical responses such as mapping, testing, and contact tracing. In another way, modernity comes with the demand for ordinary people to act as rational subjects, as understood in the secular West. For example, Ebola public health messaging often appealed to people's supposed individuality and their assumed valuing of their own life above all else and tended to underplay people's reliance on one another and social practices of care.

Modernity might figure as the solution in these narratives, but it might equally be interpreted as the root cause. Global economic expansion and industrialization over the past centuries has led to mass deforestation, urbanization, and poverty. Zoonotic diseases are now more likely than ever to transmit from animals to humans and then to spread faster and wider. Public health systems globally are widely underfunded and barely functioning, especially in former colonies and places of economic extraction such as Sierra Leone. Digging a little deeper, it is clear that the two worlds—the modern and the not—are not really distinct in the first place. Rather than the "fresh contact" implied by popular narratives of global health and, in some respects, the policy frameworks used by international actors, the worlds are in fact in deep, long-term relationship with one another. In West Africa, the story of entanglement with Western modernity is more than five hundred years old.

Ultimately, I think that the meetings I attended with international Ebola responders felt strange to me not just because they seemed at odds with my daily life in Freetown but also because these two worlds were in fact proximate and inseparably enmeshed. Several of my neighbors worked at the Radisson Blu and other hotels nearby as cleaners, porters, cooks, and receptionists. They knew this world well but from a different vantage point than the international professionals with whom I now sat. While to most Freetown residents Europe and America are foreign, described as *yanda* (over there), they are also familiar places in the social and cultural landscape. Many of my neighbors had relatives and friends who had migrated overseas but remained socially and materially important in the lives of Freetown residents, and many young people plan their own attempts to emigrate. The music, movies, and fashion of Freetown's young generations remain heavily inspired by transatlantic Black culture. The formal institutions of state and economy and school curriculums are products of British colonialism.

Freetown has deep cosmopolitan roots going back to the first group of former slaves from London who settled there at the end of the eighteenth century. And yet, among the city's ordinary residents there is a recurring pattern of neglect, of being marginal actors who are only partly and contingently included in the story of modernity. The city's cultures have continually mediated between the shifting contours of the local and the foreign. Ebola was only the latest in a string of major interventions via Freetown's large natural harbor that have defined the city's history. For Freetown's residents, economic openings, the establishing and maintenance of families and homes, and notions of agency and dependence have long been bound up with and brokered through the global forces that moved through the city.

The Houses That Molay and Foday Built

Foday, whom we met in the introduction, was my first host in the Congo Town neighborhood. He was in his early to mid-twenties at the time of the Ebola emergency. Although his life and social world had some of the hallmarks of the lost generation of disconnected youths we often read about in contemporary African cities—and to be sure, some the challenges he faced are unique to his generation—he was in fact closely following on from his parents and grandparents in attempting to build a meaningful life that straddled the close-knit social worlds of their home village in the rural Northern Province of Sierra Leone and the coastal capital city of Freetown. The Freetown in which Foday's grandfather Molay arrived in the 1950s was a different and smaller place from the bustling and sprawling city of today, but his basic projects of building a life and a family by navigating between coexisting social orders was in many ways the same.

Foday was a charismatic and good-looking young man who worked as a taxi driver. However, he was increasingly focusing on his dream to be a recording artist and a music producer. We were originally introduced by my brother Jacob, who had become close to Foday's family while living and working in Freetown. When I arrived to undertake fieldwork, Foday agreed to host me in his small two-room home, which he shared at the time with two of his cousins. All three were in their twenties.

At first glance, the surroundings of the house, near the base of the Congo River valley, could easily be described as a slum and its inhabitants as the "marginal youths" who make up a large percentage of the population of Africa's contemporary cities. The house was without running water, and electricity was sporadic. The land was a few meters above the base of a valley that flooded each rainy season, leaving all the houses around Foday's susceptible to heavy damage each year (figure 2). Foday's external walls were built with cement blocks and were therefore more secure than neighboring houses constructed from corrugated metal. As unmarried young men, none of the residents cooked regularly. Instead, they relied on neighbors and family for food or would walk to the junction with the main road to buy street food when they had some money to spend.

Yet, by the standards of young people in Freetown, Foday's situation was desirable. Despite the lack of basic amenities, his home was fitted with a TV, a sound system, a personal computer, a mixer, a keyboard and a microphone for recording music, and a dresser full of fashionable clothes. Singers and producers would regularly come to the house to record Krio- and English-language tracks inspired by American hip-hop, Nigerian afrobeat, and Jamaican dancehall.[3] The land that Foday built the house on had belonged to his now-deceased grandfather, Molay, who had passed it onto his fourth wife. Foday's grandmother was Molay's third wife, however, and there many siblings, cousins, aunts, and uncles above him in the pecking order. It was something of a coup that he managed to build on the land even if the arrangement was not favorable. The house

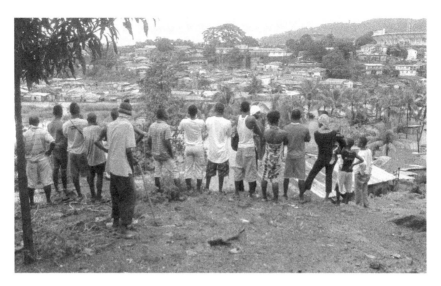

FIGURE 2.   Freetown residents observe seasonal flooding.

was leased from Molay's fourth wife, and in six years it would be handed over to her unless Foday started paying rent at that point.

Molay grew up in a Loko-speaking village in the Northern Province of the country. He had migrated to Freetown in the late 1950s as part of a large wave of rural-urban migration. As with many young migrants, he found work on the docks. Freetown had one of the largest ports along the Atlantic coast of Africa. It was used to export iron ore and other raw materials sourced in the region and also had long-held strategic significance for the Royal Navy. It was for this reason that Freetown was made the capital of British West Africa during the colonial period. With his salary, Molay was able to buy a sizable plot of land in the Congo Town area that stretched from the top to the base of the valley. At the top of the plot of land at a well-located corner of one of the streets that cuts through the neighborhood, Molay built a family compound. The compound, which remains structurally unchanged today, is divided into four two-room units, one for each wife. Foday had grown up in one of these units along with three sisters. The roof is now rusted, with holes covered by makeshift plastic bags and metal sheets. The paint has faded, and the walls are crumbling.

Yet, Molay's house remains the family hub in Freetown. Its endurance coexists with its overcrowding and crumbling facade, as subsequent generations have made it their home there in the absence of alternatives. As Foday's older brother Alhassan once explained to me, the fact that the family was not able to maintain the home or build another floor above, as other neighbors had done, is testament to the inability of family members to get along with one another and cooperate. Foday's home, in contrast to that of his grandfather, was only meant to be temporary. It was the hub not of an intergenerational family but rather of his cousins, friends, and fellow musicians, fitted with modern electronics and entertainment systems. The waged formal work that Molay and many of his generation participated in has become increasingly hard to come by. Foday's income came from informal enterprise in music and transport and from the patronage of family and friends in Freetown and overseas. His possessions and assets, the vehicle that he operated and the equipment at home, were transitory. Some were borrowed or on loan. Others would be sold when money was needed.

The family that Molay had bought the land from in the Congo Town neighborhood were Krio, the Freetown-based ethnic group that traces its history to the former slaves who had migrated from London, British colonies in the Americas, and along Africa's Atlantic coast. The neighborhood owes its name to early settlers who came indirectly from Congo via intercepted slave ships after the British ban on the international slave trade. As Fyfe, in his colorful eight hundred–page *History of Sierra Leone*, published in 1962, tells it, "The Congo people who, it is said, preferred to live by the waterside, left their hilltop at New Cabenda and followed the pretty stream dignified as the Congo River down to Whiteman's Bay where in 1816 they bought from a Maroon woman a site for a new home, Congo Town."[4]

The "pretty stream" is now part of the densely settled community where Foday built his house, and Whiteman's Bay is now a bustling port for small-scale fishing and transport and a produce market. Today there are about twenty thousand residents living in the Congo Town neighborhood. Across the valley is the Siaka Stevens national stadium, built by Chinese contractors in the 1980s. The neighborhood contains many standard features of Freetown neighborhoods, including a cemetery with its own paved access road adorned by colonial-era lampposts. The road to the cemetery, laid down shortly after independence, is the only paved road in the neighborhood. The neighborhood also includes schools, churches, mosques, small food shops and bars, tailors, makeshift workshops of carpenters and mechanics, "cinemas" for watching international football games, a covered market, and a police station. Some of the original two-story wooden Krio houses remain, built in an architectural style inspired by town houses in Louisiana and South Carolina and complete with shutter windows, wooden staircases, verandas, and attic rooms under triangular roofs.

But like most of Freetown, which has tripled in size in the last few decades, the neighborhood is much more crowded today.[5] Most of the residents are either rural migrants who began to arrive from the early 2000s in the aftermath of the civil war or are related to or descended from earlier migrants, such as Molay.

The neighborhood streets are not merely the means of moving through the neighborhood but are also spaces of business and socialization in which the distinction between "family" and "neighbor" is regularly blurred.[6] Sitting on chairs outside shops and food stalls, friends "keep time." Mechanics use corners for repairing vehicles. Children play street games, including football with goals made of rocks. Women get their hair "planted," often on a weekly basis, in makeshift street salons or by friends and sisters. Most homes do not have kitchens; cooking takes place on the veranda or in the street.

The streets are also stages for seasonal and national festivities as well as family rites of passage. In December, streets host their own carnivals in which large sound systems are leased to play through the night. Secret societies hold masquerade performances, often unannounced, on street corners. In this multifaith neighborhood of Christians and Muslims, religious festivities also take place on the street. On "pray day" (Eid), public spaces such as football fields are packed with worshippers wearing newly tailored clothes. On New Year and Easter, residents march behind their local *debul* (masquerade "devil"), who acts as a kind of neighborhood mascot. Weddings and funerals also involve processions through the streets, and the more prominent the family the bigger the procession, which in some cases includes marching bands and convoys of jeeps. Baby-naming ceremonies, in Krio called *pulnador* (take outside) are, by definition, held on the street outside the home.

Molay's generation of young immigrants was documented by the anthropologist Michael Banton in his influential book *West African City: A Study of Tribal Life in Freetown,* published in 1960. The study spoke to sociological debates, popular at the time, around "de-tribalization," which connected to the mass rural-urban migrations that were occurring around the globe. In Freetown, Banton observed new ways of being "tribal" by forming professional associations and new forms of kinship and electing tribal headmen. In other words, migrants were discovering ways of maintaining ethnic traditions and ties through distinctly modern social and political organizational forms. Additionally, rural migrants emulated the long-standing Krio political and professional class of Freetown for whom Western education and British cultural orientation were intermixed with maintaining close-knit familial networks, in part through the celebration of family rituals, particularly funerals.[7]

More recent studies of African cities, especially those centering around today's youths, tell a radically different story. In the so-called neoliberal African city, breakdown, improvisation, flexibility, and the spectral are operative concepts as economic decline, state decay, and crumbling urban infrastructure have become commonplace.[8] Rural youths continue to flock to cities in search of opportunity or after being displaced through conflict or appropriation of land, while at the same time centralized provisions for urban management deplete. Recent studies of Freetown have focused on its wartime and postwar dimensions, in which violent and neoliberal regimes of work, combined with patrimonial politics, are key organizing principles.[9] Such renderings resonate with what I saw in Freetown, but they do not tell the whole story.

The young people I got to know well and lived with certainly experienced a great deal of unpredictability and volatility in their lives, paradoxically combined with the stuckedness attributed to recent generations of poor African youths.[10] Formal health systems are badly resourced, with many people relying on informal clinics and home-based care. Jobs are hard to come by. Linked to this is the shrinking of state capacity, as the economy has radically informalized and the state, particularly the police force, has become actively predatory regarding vulnerable young informal workers. Intimate and familial relationships are marked by monetary indebtedness, giving them great potential for instability as boundaries blur between friends, rivals, business partners, debtors, creditors, family, and housemates. The international world is often seen as the only real way out through out-migration or financial flows from diasporic remittances and NGO development programs.

However, the world that I knew in the Congo Town neighborhood did not fit neatly into the more apocalyptic paradigms of African city life, even if the constituent elements were there. These elements coexisted with more structured types of associational and family organization described in their nascent forms in mid-twentieth century accounts of the city. It is even possible that dependence on these forms of support has increased now that the workplace and the state cannot be relied on as they once could. There is a strong community ethos in Freetown neighborhoods and a high degree of secular and religious associational membership. The looser individualized subjectivities associated with contemporary neoliberal cultures and the anonymities of cosmopolitan city living are balanced with the close-knit neighborly lifestyles. While the young men such as Foday at the heart of this book might at times resemble the hustlers and "shifters" inhabiting the African megacity, much of their social lives center around less glamorous and desperate, albeit contentious, arenas of family and domestic life, arenas largely unaccounted for in renderings of contemporary African cities.[11] The children and grandchildren of migrants to Freetown maintain strong connections both to family in their home villages and family members who have migrated overseas. Banton might have been interested to know that Foday and his siblings still considered Molay's birthplace "their village." Foday would visit several times a year for festive occasions as well as when he was unwell to be looked after by his mother and father who returned there after decades in Freetown.

In the sections below, I outline three aspects of Sierra Leone's globally inter-connected history that are particularly significant in the shaping of the region today: slavery, colonialism, and independence. In times of emergency, it is as if buried, traumatic histories erupt from below the surface, playing out again in new, unsettling configurations. The key point, though, is that the Ebola epidemic and the international and local responses did not come out of nowhere. While old disruptive dynamics of foreign intervention were replayed during the emergency, the integration of long histories of global entanglement mean that frameworks were in place through which ordinary people caught up in the Ebola emergency were able to respond in their own terms. As with Foday and his grandfather Mo-lay, strategies for dealing with the imbalances between different social orders have been passed down through the generations.

Slavery

The Atlantic slave trade, in which over ten million enslaved Africans were shipped to the Americas between the sixteenth and nineteenth centuries, was central in shaping the world today and, not least, Sierra Leone. The country's name is a variation of Serra Lyoa (Lioness Mountain), coined by a Portuguese explorer in 1462 with reference to the shape of the mountains along the Free-town peninsula. As in much of West Africa, trade in commodities such as ivory and gold developed along the coastal areas and down rivers. Gradually expand-ing trade networks significantly impacted the organization of local societies. The region's thick forests and coastline are thought to have separated from others in precolonial times. Yet, not long after European contact, parallel and likely con-nected radical transformations were taking place inland with the Mane inva-sions from the north, ultimately linked to the spread of Islam. By the mid-sixteenth century the region had become well integrated into the Atlantic system in which British companies and forces dominated.

Extractive trade relationships emerged over a period of centuries, but a major turning point was the sheer scale of the trade in people that comprised the Atlan-tic slave trade. From 1562, demands for labor in the colonized lands of the Amer-icas fueled the capture and transportation of West Africans who would then be sold into slavery. Investments came from loans from grossers in the city of Lon-don, who funded private shipping and slaving operations based in British port cities such as Bristol, Liverpool, and Southampton. In what is known as the trian-gular trade, slaves were shipped from Africa to the Americas, coffee and sugar was shipped from the Americas to Europe, and arms and textiles and other manufactured goods were shipped from Europe to Africa. Sierra Leone was one of the primary sites of capture in West Africa, particularly for slaves bound for North America. Linguistic and cultural connections to Sierra Leone can be observed to this day among the Gullah people, the African America group living in the Low Country region of Florida, Georgia, and South Carolina. Many African Americans trace their family back to a slaving castle at Bunce Island in the Sierra Leone River, which has become a tourism and pilgrimage site in recent years.

The Atlantic slave trade had a major impact on social formations around the coast of Africa and farther inland.[12] Low-density internal slavery coexisted with the high-density slavery of the Atlantic trade. Unlike high-density slaves, who were permanent social outsiders used purely as labor, low-density slaves were varyingly incorporated into local kinship systems. In some cases, slaves had their own social units that, while distinct from full households, reproduced kinship-like structures over time in tandem with full households. In African contexts, slaves sometimes held positions of political power, in part because they were not seen as threats to those who were freeborn. In other cases, slaves did marry into elite lineages. The huge demand for slaves during the Atlantic trade led to a new class of local "big men," who gained power by brokering between European traders and traditional authorities. The trade, however, encouraged raiding and conflict between political groups. Times of crisis would often see shifts in internal slavery from low density to high density.[13]

Internal slavery in West Africa came to a "slow death."[14] Slavery was legal in most of Sierra Leone beyond Freetown until 1927, more than a century after the ban of the international trade. British colonial authorities relied on slave labor economically and were willing to tolerate and even quietly encourage it even if they claimed to promote abolitionism. Historians have linked the demise of legal slavery to a number of factors, including the economic collapse of the Great Depression as well as the resistance of slaves after returning from fighting in World War I.

However, the boundaries between the practices of internal slavery and kinship-based dependencies in Sierra Leone have continued to be blurry. On the one hand, kinship has long represented liberation from slavery, as slaves secure their rights over children and spouses in some cases through the payment of bride prices. And yet, on the other hand, incorporation into kinship groups on unfavorable terms is itself often understood as a form of enslavement. In agrarian economies in rural Sierra Leone and in West Africa more broadly, labor is traditionally scarcer than land, so economic power has been understood as connected less to the ownership of land, money, and things and more to "wealth in people."[15] "Big men" typically accumulate wealth in people by marrying their daughters to young men who are unable to pay bride prices. They are thus forced to work the land of their fathers-in-law to pay off their debt. The dissatisfaction of rural youths with such exploitative relationships was a driving cause in many leaving their villages and joining rebel groups during the civil war in the late twentieth century. Even in Freetown today, young people who feel stuck in exploitative domestic relationships describe their predicament as slavery.

If the mass extraction and commodification of people is one side of the story of the Atlantic salve trade, then the founding of Freetown is another. Freetown was settled in 1787 by four hundred or so former slaves from London. The land was bought from a local king by the London-based Committee for the Relief of the Black Poor. The early settlers faced poor harvests, conflict with neighboring groups, and an attack by French sailors. With limited options, some of the settlers worked for local slavers or established their own slaving operations. With the momentum of abolitionism growing after decades of grassroots campaigning and resistance, the slave trade in the British Empire was formally banned by an act of Parliament in 1807, although the practice of slavery in many British colonies remained legal. Prior to this, Thomas Peters, the African-born campaigner who had escaped slavery in America, held meetings with abolitionists in London and the Sierra Leone Company, who agreed that Freetown would be formally designated as a refuge for freed slaves. Peters led a second wave of settlers, known as "black loyalists," who came via Nova Scotia. They had escaped from plantations in Virginia and South Carolina and gained freedom after fighting for the British in the American Revolutionary War. Subsequent waves of settlers included Jamaican Maroons and a piecemeal migration of Black British colonial subjects, particularly those who had fought in the Napoleonic Wars. Many additional recaptives, slaves intercepted from illegal slaving operations, were sent to Freetown, despite originating from sometimes distant parts of the continent. By 1850, Freetown's population had risen to fifty thousand.

Colonialism

The multifaceted history of slavery in Sierra Leone cannot be understood beyond the colonial structures in which it was enmeshed. Freetown was ceded to form a British crown colony in 1808—only thirty years after it was founded as a refuge for former slaves—and served as the capital of British West Africa. Freetown's sizable natural harbor was a well-suited base for the Royal Navy as well as a port for the export of agricultural and mineral resources. Throughout the nineteenth century, the colony expanded from Freetown and its immediate vicinity into the interior of Sierra Leone, increasing British access to commerce and resources. By the late nineteenth century, Britain faced increasing competition with France over regional influence in what came to be known as the "scramble for Africa."

The British employed their preferred method of indirect rule in colonizing the interior of Sierra Leone. Instead of institutionalizing a state bureaucracy and a legal system throughout the territory, the British acquired economic and political control by developing favorable patronage relationships with preexisting or newly created "customary" elites. Freetown residents, particularly the Krios—the ethnic group who trace their lineage to the city's transatlantic formerly enslaved founders and settlers—were cast as mediators between Indigenous groups and Europeans, negotiating treaties and trade agreements. This role led to both socioeconomic prominence within the colonial hierarchy and racist resentment by colonial authorities. While the positions of the Krio people in Sierra Leonean society has shifted over the centuries, they represent an enduring model for brokerage between local and global social orders for Freetown residents of different ethnic backgrounds.

In 1896 the British established the Sierra Leone Protectorate, which encompassed much of the country today. Despite its name, the protectorate utilized forceful and coercive measures. Few "native" authorities subjugated themselves to the British willingly. Many organized armed resistance against colonial authorities, most famously the chief Bai Bureh, leader of the Hut Tax War who is depicted on one of Sierra Leone's banknotes. Existing political structures were replaced with a network of "paramount chiefs," local authorities who were pliable to British interest. The paramount chieftaincy system is still in place today. The expansion of imperial influence from the crown colony of Freetown to the protectorate came hand in hand with a reverse migration of people from the interior to the coastal city. While some became involved in the production and export of agricultural products—palm oil, cocoa beans, and coffee as well as raw materials such as iron ore and, later, bauxite and diamonds—the majority of the residents of the protectorate engaged in small-scale farming of cassava, rice, and peanuts as well as hunting and fishing.

The colony, comprising Freetown and its immediate surroundings, and the protectorate, the vast mostly rural hinterland of Sierra Leone, were separated only by an invisible boundary. Yet, each had its own separate legal and administrative systems, which remain distinct today. Colony residents were subjects of the British Crown and were therefore required to abide by English law, whereas protectorate residents were subject to the customary law of native courts and the "improvised justice" of the Frontier Police. Land tenure in the colony operated with English concepts of freehold interest, while those of the protectorate were rooted in customary principles.[16] While slavery was banned in the colony in the early nineteenth century, it was legal in the protectorate until the twentieth century.

Christopher Fyfe's *History of Sierra Leone* is dotted with a litany of accounts of deadly epidemics during the British colonial period for which the mosquito-

ridden marshes and jungles around the Freetown peninsula were a natural breed-
ing ground. For the year 1859, Fyfe notes:

> One disease after another broke out—fever, yellow fever, measles. Small-
> pox ravaged the villages [around Freetown]. At least 500 died in seven
> months. The doctors fell ill, Dr Bradshaw, the Colonial Surgeon, with
> yellow fever—from which, a rare case, he recovered. Only one Army
> Surgeon was left to tend the sick. The forty-two European deaths (half
> the European population) included both bishops, the Roman Catholic
> priests, and the headmaster of the Grammar School and his wife. Only
> one senior official died, Smyth, the Colonial Secretary, of smallpox.
> It was in this terrible year that the vultures or turkey-buzzards are
> said to have first come to Freetown where they have since been so
> conspicuous.[17]

There were other major yellow fever outbreaks in 1884, 1897, and 1916.[18] Options to drain the swampy regions at the turn of the century were discounted,
with the Colonial Office finally opting to move Europeans to the hills, which
were served by a newly built railway line. The expression "white man's grave"
was coined in popular colonial-era accounts of West Africa.

The White colonialists were, of course, much better off than most of Freetown's Black residents. British colonial approaches to disease management tended
to be authoritarian and punitive. They employed techniques such as quarantining and disease mapping, measures that were central to the official Ebola response in 2014–2016.[19] The effectiveness of colonial-era public health measures
were undermined by the little attention given to caregiving and material support for the poor and sick. By far the deadliest epidemic to hit Sierra Leone was
the global 1918 influenza pandemic, known as the Spanish flu, that killed fifty
million people worldwide and at least hundreds of thousands in West Africa.
The virus entered Freetown through the harbor and then spread via the thousands of dockworkers and ultimately along train lines and other trade routes into
the interior, devastating communities throughout the country.[20] The death toll
from the flu and from the food shortages connected to it was a significant
factor in growing dissatisfaction with colonial governance, along with the mass
recruitment of young men to fight in World War I.[21]

The position of the Krio people shifted radically during the twentieth century.
As mentioned above, the ethnic group inhabited a political and economic niche
as mediators between native groups and the British colonizers. The Krio legal
status was nonnative, that is, not belonging to any of the country's sixteen ethnic groups. The Krio people were somewhat assimilated into British colonial
culture, expressed in involvement in education, forms of property ownership,

English-sounding names, Western dress, transatlantic architectural styles, Christian religious practice, and links to the Black diaspora. In a new constitution drafted in 1951, the protectorate and the colony were formally united after much contestation and resistance from Krio authorities. As White colonial officials took over as middlemen, Krio people found themselves on the receiving end of increasingly direct racism. At the same time, a new cohort of political elites from native ethnic groups began to replace Krio politicians, taking advantage of their ties with residents in the former protectorate. However, Krio businessmen retained control of economic niches in the capital, while others acted as influential members of Freetown's professional and civil society. The Krio people developed more covert and performative means of maintaining their elite status while emphasizing their distinctiveness from other Sierra Leoneans.[22]

Postcolony and Conflict

Sierra Leone gained national independence in 1961. Unlike the more anticolonial and revolutionary breaks in other former colonies in Africa, such as Ghana and Kenya, and in neighboring Guinea, Sierra Leone's independence was markedly conservative. Sierra Leone has continued to be Western-leaning and procapitalist in its orientation, with political relations maintained with its former colonizer. An important factor was the country's sizable economic growth in the period directly preceding independence. The 1950s saw growth in diamond and iron ore mining. This funded infrastructural developments, such as roads, railways, and schools and colleges.[23]

In 1968 after a democratic transition of power between political parties and two failed military coups, Siaka Stevens came into office, initiating over two decades of what was in effect a one-party state. Faced with the inherited dual system of government of elected representatives in urban areas and the chieftaincy systems in rural areas, an informal network of patrimonialism thrived in place of formal political and economic processes. The global economic crises in the 1970s, fueled by the skyrocketing price of oil, hit Sierra Leone hard, as occurred with many economies in the Global South. The state in its weak neopatrimonial form was ill-equipped to respond effectively, while international arrangements effectively negated any alternative. Sierra Leone, like most poor states under Euro-American capitalist influence, underwent major structural adjustment reforms from the 1970s to 1990s, which attempted to loosen the state's grip on the free market. In hindsight, it is clear that these policies amounted to little more than weakening any political and economic obstacles to the continued extraction of resources and wealth from the Global South to the Global North while maintaining favorable market conditions for importing foreign goods, such as by cutting local trade tariffs. In 1979 the International Monetary Fund negotiated an economic stabilization plan for Sierra Leone, loaning the government money under the condition that it reduce state spending. Major cuts were made in the areas of infrastructure, manufacturing, health, and education. The railways were permanently closed, along with a major iron ore mine. The economy subsequently collapsed, with drastic shortages of staple foods, and roughly 80 percent of the population falling below the poverty line. Political and economic elites in Sierra Leone began to prioritize their own short-term security—supplying imported rice to clients such as the army and the police—over long-term survival by, for example, employing and supporting the education of their loyal subjects.[24]

Long-term prospects looked poor as Sierra Leone's financial dependency on external organizations and countries increased, with economic arrangements turning increasingly extractive. This sowed the seeds for the decade-long civil war, beginning in 1991, following a military coup led by a twenty-six-year-old junior officer, Valentine Strasser, in response to a recent "democratic" election that was understood to be rigged. International pressure mounted to overthrow Strasser, who posed a threat to the existing economic and political arrangements. International sanctions on trade brought the country's economy to the breaking point. The war itself was a spillover from Charles Taylor's uprising in neighboring Liberia. In Sierra Leone, rebel groups were led by the Revolutionary United Front (RUF), composed of an alliance between young, educated revolutionaries dissatisfied with the failing political and economic system and mainly uneducated rural youths escaping harsh labor conditions cemented by forced marriages and indebtedness to local elders. The RUF fought a stealthy guerrilla war primarily out of camps in the rainforest but also took major regional towns and parts of Freetown. The RUF employed shock tactics, such as extreme and performative violence, but was also driven by neoliberal logics of "just in time" economic production.[25] The underpaid military proved unable to contain the RUF, and the use of external mercenaries by the government was financially unsustainable. In the late 1990s following the second rebel invasion of Freetown, British and Nigerian military intervened. The RUF came under increasing financial pressure as trading links to Liberia became strained and in 2001 signed a peace accord. An estimated two million people were displaced during the war, many of them youths.

The closing stages of the war and its aftermath saw the deployment of international peacekeepers, a World Bank–sponsored disarmament, demobilization, and reintegration program aimed at the former rebel soldiers and a high-profile liberal peace and reconciliation process operating out of Freetown.[26] During the Ebola state of emergency, international and state militaries were again deployed on the ground, with the official response taking on a highly securitized flavor as military checkpoints were set up countrywide. The postwar period saw a proliferation of NGO-centered development and humanitarian activity—described as the "crisis caravan"[27]—focusing on areas such as youth empowerment, family planning, and disease prevention. Some successes were achieved in the management of cholera, Lassa fever, and HIV/AIDS and in restarting vaccination programs. However, the aid industry's reliance on international funding contributed to failings in several areas. Funding disproportionally targeted "exceptional" viruses such as HIV, with programs poorly integrated with efforts to address wider societal and public health failings.[28] The relatively rapid turnover of international staff working in the aid sector of Sierra Leone in the postwar years meant that when Ebola hit, there were limited numbers who had experience in working in Sierra Leone's public sector.[29] In addition, the security of international staff in aid organizations was prioritized over those in impacted communities, reproducing global, racialized health hierarchies.[30]

The international aid apparatus has become an ordinary part of the hustle and bustle of life in Freetown and many other towns and cities in the region, albeit in a smaller-scale form than during emergencies such as Ebola. Public health posters appear around the town, along with NGOs' signs, branded gear, and white jeeps. International NGO jobs are widely coveted by workers in Freetown due to the pay and benefits they offer. NGO talk has infused the everyday language, while numerous local development and youth empowerment groups offer NGO-inspired sensitization programs and development initiatives.

In 2007, a relatively peaceful general election was held in which there was an internationally celebrated democratic transfer of power from the Sierra Leone People's Party to the All People's Congress. And in 2018, the reverse occurred. Yet, Sierra Leone remains one of the poorest countries in the world. There is widespread dissatisfaction with the political process, with continual reports of corrupt practices, political infighting, and a disconnect between mainstream political discourse and the reality on the ground. State-sponsored development projects, increasingly outsourced to Chinese companies, are regarded as superficial and short-term initiatives, rarely contributing to meaningful local investment, as the country's natural resources are routinely signed off to foreign investors in shortsighted deals. Popular personal engagement with the state, through its legal and bureaucratic institutions and medical facilities, is often fraught, regularly relying on informal arrangements or bribes, with state employees being routinely underpaid. Young people are still faced with limited economic opportunities, relying on precarious informal work to get by or the support of patrons, family, and friends with means. Health systems are highly underdeveloped and actually de-developed in line with the neoliberal doctrine of recent decades that has seen international demands for state expenditures to be cut. Infant and maternal mortality rates are among the highest globally. These conditions sowed the seeds for Ebola to become not only a regional emergency in Sierra Leone and its neighboring countries of Guinea and Liberia but also, in the language of the World Health Organization, a public health emergency of international concern, paving the way for another large-scale, narrowly focused international intervention.

In 2014–2016, Ebola represented both a deadly affliction and a large-scale public health and humanitarian intervention. The emergency was in many ways a manifestation of the very precarities that have characterized ordinary life in poor African cities such as Freetown. The infectious disease thrived in crowded communities that lack adequate health and sanitation infrastructure and in places where the state and other bureaucratic entities are either mistrusted or absent. But at the same time, as the following chapters will reveal, the time of emergency was not unfamiliar and, in surprising ways, was widely welcomed by young Freetown residents as a period of unusual clarity and possibility. As opposed to the notion of two worlds embedded in global health discourse, the language of international intervention was neither alien nor unintelligible to ordinary people in Freetown. Rather, it was like a dialect of their own cosmopolitan language.

Freetown and many other cities in the Global South have been modern for hundreds of years, a fact that is repeatedly forgotten. Many of the customs and organizational forms of the Krio elite from the early and mid-twentieth century, who were culturally and socially interconnected with British colonial and Black transatlantic culture, have become mainstream in Freetown among the non-Krio majority. The intertwining of professional and familial networks, renegotiated around ritual occasions, has become widespread. Brokerage between local and global social orders remains a primary means of economic gain and social mobility in the spheres of work and family.[31] Kinship in Freetown has long toed a blurry line between slavery and freedom, which young people such as Foday continue to navigate to this day.

In making sense of and responding to the Ebola emergency, Freetown residents were conditioned by the everyday social, economic, and political entanglements immediately preceding and during the outbreak. But they also drew upon deeper personal and societal memory: the experiences of crisis and intervention during and after the civil war in the 1990s and early 2000s, the legacies of British colonialism and independence, and the largely buried history of the slave trade, of which the coastal areas around Freetown were primary locations of extraction and trade of human cargo as well sites of freedom and return. This history is essential to understanding why an underresourced and vulnerable state with a highly depleted medical infrastructure was yet again so susceptible to heavy-handed foreign intervention and equally, how residents of Freetown, a poor yet historically cosmopolitan city, were equipped to shape how it played out in their own terms.

HAZARD PAY

One morning I received a disturbing phone call from a young man known as Human Right. The previous night he was involved in a serious accident on his motorbike and was in desperate need of medical attention. A traffic policeman standing by the side of the road had gestured for him to pull over. Human Right swerved out the way, and the policeman grabbed onto him. Human Right came flying off his bike and landed on an exposed iron rod, which penetrated his groin, narrowly missing his testicles. Human Right spent the night in a crowded cell while his injury went untreated.

Human Right was the self-given nickname of a taxi driver in his late twenties. He worked for Foday and a number of other taxi operators in the neighborhood, which had become like a second home to him. Human Right would normally crash with friends or sleep in the car, but recently he had been staying at his apprentice's place. The apprentice, known by his own nickname, Balloon Burst, had a small room near his family compound. I was friendly with both, and they would regularly invite me to ride along with them.

Human Right had a reputation for being something of a free agent. He was a technically gifted and confident driver who knew every backroad in town. He would find miraculous gaps in traffic jams, maneuver around impossibly tight corners, and traverse streets that, in the rainy season, were more river than road. While driving passengers, he loved to give informal lecturers, full of street slang, on topics such as Rastafarian spirituality, national politics, entrepreneurialism, and Christian morality. Human Right's family lived in the East End (or "East Coast," as he liked to call it), and he would visit them most days that he was working, along with friends dotted around town. Although he relied on the "fast money" he earned on the road, the actual job of taxi driving never really felt like Human Right's primary motivation; it was more a vehicle for self-expression and maintaining social relationships strung across the city.

Human Right began working on the streets at age fourteen, when he dropped out of school because of financial hardship faced by his parents. His father, who once enjoyed a regular salary working for a shipping company, had suffered debilitating physical injuries; he now needed a crutch to walk. He had not been able to find regular work after the economy had reopened in the early 2000s after the civil war. Human Right was initially an apprentice on a *poda poda* (minibus taxi), gathering passengers and collecting money. This was a common route to becoming a driver; it was expected that drivers would teach apprentices to drive on the side. For many years now, Human Right had worked on commission for taxi operators and owners while also teaching many apprentices to drive.

Balloon Burst was Human Right's apprentice, but they had become distanced in the months preceding the accident. Balloon Burst, who shared his small room with his partner and their baby daughter, was not happy with his boss regularly staying over. So, Human Right, somewhat dejected, moved back to the East End. Things were not looking much better on the business front. It had been almost a year since he bought a taxi, a proud symbol of self-reliance. But the car was old and banged up, requiring too much maintenance for the investment to pay off. He sold the car for a small fee and bought two old motorbikes with additional money borrowed from his mother, who ran a rotating credit association with women from their church. The bikes were to be operated commercially as *okada* (motorbike taxis). But Human Right was struggling to earn enough to pay back the debt. Regulations on travel and commercial transport during the Ebola state of emergency as well as lockdowns and curfews had slowed business. "The streets are dry," Human Right told me one evening when we were driving around together.

Okada are a popular means of commercial transport in Freetown. They have the advantage of being able to climb steep unpaved roads, which are plentiful in the mountainous and rapidly growing city. Motorbikes can also weave through traffic jams in the old narrow streets downtown. Working as an okada rider is one of few options for uneducated young men to earn an income. But it is not an easy job. Accidents are not uncommon, and victimization by aggressive policing is routine.

Human Right's accident had not come out of nowhere. In fact, he had several minor mishaps on the bike in a matter of weeks. Only a few days before the accident I had received a call from Human Right's mother, who was worried about the bind that her son was in. She recalled a recent dream in which an intimidating gang of boys had come to the family home asking for Human Right. She fended them off but feared that they would find him elsewhere.

The dream was alarming on several levels. Psychologically, it spoke to a son's vulnerability and a mother's helplessness to protect him and perhaps to a mother's feelings of guilt. But the dream was also prophetic, preempting a crisis that was to come while containing echoes of traumatic history. When the rebel soldiers entered Freetown during the civil war, Human Right's family had fled from their home, taking refuge in the abandoned the Princess Christian Maternity Hospital (nicknamed "Cottage Hospital") downtown.

When I got the call the day after the accident, Balloon Burst and I traveled across town, where we met Human Right along with his distraught mother, father, and sister outside a small local pharmacy. I had often witnessed and felt the strong obligations for family and friends to come close during such moments of crisis. It was this very impulse that made Ebola at times doubly difficult. Attempts to care for friends of family in need, including in cases that had nothing directly to do with the disease, could be met with additional challenges.

It was not only Human Right's family and friends who rallied around him. Human Right also received the support from his fellow okada riders by way of the Sierra Leone Commercial Bike Riders Union (BRU). A sizable group had gathered to protest Human Right's abuse at the hands of the police, led by a union official. The case gained traction in part because it demonstrated so overtly the kind of abuse of police power that okada riders routinely experience. The group entered the police station to negotiate Human Right's release from custody and to demand that the officer who had forcibly pulled him from his bike be brought to justice. The authorities at the station, undoubtedly feeling under pressure, issued a report that entitled Human Right to medical compensation. But Human Right's family deemed the bureaucratic procedures too long-winded to enact. The family, knowing that an immediate full payment would not be necessary, decided to go to the local pharmacy to have the wound stitched up. Human Right was stoic, not showing signs of pain. We discussed making arrangements for him to come back and stay in our neighborhood again, given that his return to the East End had been so ill-fated.

Human Right's accident revealed with unusual visibility—not least through the different parties that showed up—the conflation of social, economic, and political forces that structure everyday life and work for ordinary young people in Freetown. Challenges in intimate relationships, such as between Human Right and his family and apprentice, are inseparable from financial pressures and physical dangers. In Freetown's tough informal economy, the risk of injury or death is the price demanded for sourcing an income. There is, of course, a broader and underlying political reality that the BRU protest pointed to, namely that the underresourced state apparatus is simultaneously coercive and neglectful toward ordinary workers.

Both of these characteristics—coerciveness and neglect—are embodied by Freetown's police force. Police officers are a visible presence at major junctions and roundabouts. In a crowded city with close to no traffic lights, they serve a welcome function in moving traffic along. But as I learned from my own experience of driving in Freetown (and being taught to drive there in a taxi), it does not take long to grow resentful of the traffic police. They are notorious for opportunistically extracting fines and bribes from okada riders and taxi drivers, who are both likely to have cash on hand (collected from fares) while being typically low enough in status that they pose little threat to the officers. For commercial drivers to avoid roadside abuse normally requires paying *bora*, a term used to describe traditional gifts given by youths to elders in rural settings. The ultimate casualties of coercive policing are the hundreds and more probably thousands of youths currently in Pademba Road, the city's overcrowded colonial-era prison. With most of these young inmates unable to pay bribes, fines, and (especially) lawyer's fees, they await trials that are recurringly suspended.

The police and the legal system are not, however, singularly to blame. The state does not have the available funds to maintain these institutions. Corruption by political and economic elites makes things worse, of course. But decades of international pressure by organizations such as the World Bank and the International Monetary Fund to "liberalize" the economy by cutting trade tariffs and reducing state expenditure and regulation gets more to the root of the problem. As a consequence, the police force creatively funds its operations from the bottom up rather than the top down. State neglect extends beyond the legal system. Roads are poorly maintained, and major infrastructure projects are outsourced to international companies, increasingly Chinese, thus limiting internal economic stimulus. There is no operational public transport system, despite various failed attempts to create one. Adequate health care is not readily available for informal workers. And decades of dwindling industry forces youths such as Human Right onto the streets in search of fast money.

This chapter follows commercial bike riders before and during the Ebola emergency, which provides a revealing perspective on the relationship between work, emergency, and the state. Ambivalent relationships with the state have long characterized commercial bike riding in Sierra Leone. The industry was developed by former rebel soldiers in the early 2000s but has become increasingly hierarchical and bureaucratic in its operations, despite continued conflict with the police. The Ebola state of emergency entailed new obstacles for informal workers, as described above, but also new opportunities for formal employment and recognition as tens of thousands of young people were recruited into the official

Ebola response through the hazard pay scheme. The combination of coerciveness and neglect that has characterized marginal workers' experience of the contemporary state shifted during the epidemic for these employees and others as the state took on a temporarily more bureaucratic and well-resourced form.

In this chapter, I describe the ways that marginal workers reconfigured their relationships with the state during the emergency by drawing on their experiences of work and associational life before the epidemic. The account presented here complicates dominant critiques of humanitarian and emergency responses, including Ebola, that emphasize how state and other bureaucratic entities opportunistically use crises to extend their reach and influence at the expense of ordinary people. Here in a notably urban context, grassroots organizing before Ebola was itself quite bureaucratic in form. The bureaucratized emergency response was widely welcomed by normally marginalized informal workers, while those incorporated into it were well equipped to shape the official response in their own image.

Fighting the State?

I regularly spotted an unusual character riding around the streets of Freetown on a motorbike. He looked as if he had stepped out of an old photo of the Black Panthers. He dressed from head to toe in elaborate outfits with military-style caps, shoes or boots so shiny you could see your reflection in them, black sunglasses, shiny silver buttons, an ID card holder around his neck, and a badge that read "Chief Inspector of Okada." He looked subversive, cool, and rebellious while at the same time resembling a military official–cum–civil servant. I eventually began talking to this man and discovered that he was famous among the city's commercial bike riders. He was known as Councilor.

Councilor was campaigning for the upcoming biannual bike park elections. Bike parks are administrative units of the BRU as well as physical locations where okada riders meet. There are about thirty bike parks in Freetown, and Councilor was running to become chairman of one of the largest. During his campaign he had managed to register with the union a large number of bike riders from across town, enabling them to vote for him. On the day of the election, thousands of riders gathered at a repurposed football pitch to cast their vote while Councilor rode up and down the length of the field rallying the crowd. As the hot afternoon drew on, the crowd grew restless and excited. Police, fearing a riot, arrived to disperse the gathering. Their arrival almost looked like a scripted scene in a play or movie. For one, the guns that they were purposively wielding were clearly not loaded. The votes were finally counted, and Councilor won by a

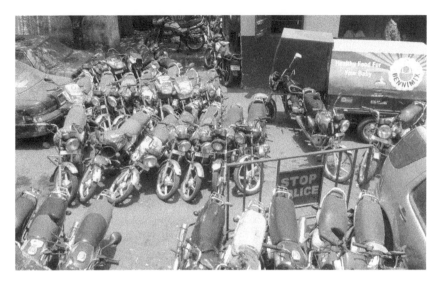

FIGURE 3.   Confiscated commercial motorbikes at a police station.

landslide. Hundreds of bikes proceeded through the streets in celebration accompanied by a cacophony of honking horns, screams, and a blasting portable sound system.

Councilor's arresting appearance—a cocktail of conformity and nonconformity—matched the way he went about his business. He rode with a briefcase sandwiched between the handlebars as he weaved through traffic, whizzing into narrow back alleys to avoid police and checkpoints. His briefcase held certificates, paperwork, pens, stamps, tape, tickets, and shoe polish. He held impromptu meetings with members of his committee in shabby roadside tea joints and bars, where he would set up a makeshift office, carefully unpacking and placing the contents of the briefcase on a table or bench.

Councilor appealed to his supporters in the union by being both "one of them," a street-savvy former rebel turned bike rider, and also an official able to use his charisma and personal (albeit unstable) relationships with police officers and politicians to bail riders and their confiscated bikes out of police custody (figure 3). Councilor was criticized, however, when the balance looked out of whack. Some labeled him "too civilian" and therefore lacking influence and also criticized his erratic behavior, while others condemned him for forgetting his "brothers" at the bike park as he advanced his personal interests.

Councilor's paradoxes were shared by the BRU as a whole. The union's discourse was steeped in the language of resistance and nonhierarchical brotherhood.[1] Rather than uniting workers against exploitation from bosses, as labor unions in the Global North typically function, the BRU saw the state as its main oppressor. And yet, the BRU itself had become a rather state-like national bureaucratic entity. Some riders saw this as inevitable and in fact as desirable. They wanted something substantial to show for their daily and annual registration fees. The union could give them legitimacy by looking like the state and forming partnerships with it, which would in practical ways alleviate the marginalization they experienced at the hands of the police and the legal system. The union had recently established its own internal police force, known as a task force, that wore a uniform of blue one shade lighter than that of the police.[2] The union also promised to hire its own lawyers and health care workers to serve its members.

Other state-like qualities of the BRU included the opportunity it gave its members to participate in a democratic, bureaucratic, political process. By contrast, as many young people in Sierra Leone do not hold national ID cards, they are unable to vote in national elections. Nor do they tend to see the state and elected governments as genuinely serving their own interests. But the union could easily fall short of its billing. The question that was always hovering over it was whether the union really served its members or instead had become an equally exploitative version or even an arm of the state. This question felt particularly pressing to me when I saw the BRU's uniformed task force physically manhandling riders who were not respecting traffic regulations.

Ambivalence to the state has characterized commercial bike riding in Sierra Leone since its inception. Motorbikes have been used as a means of rural transport for a number of decades. They are well suited for traversing dirt roads and bush paths that connect towns and villages. The availability of affordable bikes, typically imported from India via neighboring Guinea, allowed the okada industry to grow in towns and cities in the aftermath of the civil war. Commercial bike riding initially took off in former rebel strongholds, such as the regional urban centers of Makeni and Bo. Funding came indirectly from the disarmament, demobilization, and reintegration program that was enacted between 1999 and 2004 by the government of Sierra Leone with the support of the World Bank and a variety of NGOs. The program, which reached seventy-two thousand combatants, involved the exchange of weapons for money as well as skills training in such areas as carpentry and engineering. By far the most popular profession to emerge from the program, however, was informal commercial bike riding, as many ex-combatants traded their packages in motorbikes.[3] As the industry spread, so too did riding associations. Okada riding took off in Freetown in the mid-2000s, growing significantly over the decade to come. Initially major towns and urban districts were represented by their own associations; three formed in Freetown itself. In 2006, these were amalgamated to form a Freetown-wide association named One Brother. In late 2007 after meetings in Makeni, an interim national-level association was established in which bylaws and a constitution were drafted. In the same year the national Traffic Regulation Act was signed, which included sections on safety standards for bikes and protocols for formally licensing bikes as commercial vehicles with their own distinctive number plates. In 2010, the BRU became an officially recognized association by the government. Union officials described this to me as the apex in their fluctuating relationship with the state.

In 2013 relations between the BRU and the state once again became tense, as I witnessed firsthand. The government initiated a high-profile, image-conscious program to clear bike riders from Freetown's central business district altogether. This was problematic for bike riders, as it not only restricted their market but also effectively severed the eastern and western parts of town from one another. The state used increasingly stringent measures, such as the deployment of military police, armed with large batons, at major junctions. The fines and bribes that police routinely imposed on riders—to either avoid arrest or facilitate the release of a rider or a bike—increased by about tenfold. Bike riders, such as those who rallied around Human Right after his accident, grew resentful.

And then in 2014, Ebola hit. A state of emergency was declared, and international agencies linked up with national political structures in constituting the official Ebola response. The state of emergency was, on one level, bad news for bike riders. Lockdowns, curfews, and regulations on travel all contributed to a shrinking transport market. The state in some departments was more empowered to act in an executive manner. After the Ebola state of emergency was lifted in 2016, the former minister of defense turned head of the National Ebola Response Centre was tasked with overseeing the regulation of commercial transport in Freetown.

But decline and conflict do not tell whole story. For many bike riders—and young Freetown residents in general—the Ebola state of emergency, in perhaps surprising ways, represented a less predatory and more fair manifestation of the state, particularly in comparison to what they had become used to in recent years. It was not that the deeply grooved patterns of marginalization and exploitation disappeared overnight, but rather that the novel emergency bureaucratic structures were not yet fully tainted with the patterns of exclusion that those at the bottom were accustomed to. New financial flows in the form of humanitarian assistance and aid created rare openings for salaried work and formal employment. Tens of thousands of young people joined the state payroll as Ebola responders in the hazard pay scheme. This was a far cry from what most bike riders had thought possible, and yet such an ideal of formality had persisted through decades of economic decline and informalization.

The layered history of commercial bike riding and the BRU helps us understand how an international bureaucratic emergency response came to be welcomed by many of those who were incorporated into it. It was not simply that opportunities came out of nowhere, although the multibillion-dollar international intervention is partly what made them possible. Rather, there was a latent potential for formality in long-standing associational structures that informal workers were actively engaged with. This tendency became realized in new configurations of work during the emergency alongside a tendency for improvisation and adaptation, in particular due to the fact that new jobs would last only as long as the epidemic was recognized as a global threat.

Ebola Money

Peter, an okada rider who worked closely with Councilor, held the official title of "public relations officer" on the bike park committee that Councilor chaired. Fittingly, I found Peter easy to talk with, and we would meet up regularly. He was much more educated than most okada riders, although he did not come from a particularly privileged background. When he was not working as a bike rider and engaged in BRU matters, he was studying for an undergraduate degree at Fourah Bay College, Freetown's historic university. As with a large number of bike riders and other informal workers, Peter was recruited into the official Ebola response through the government hazard pay scheme.

Peter was first posted to transport medical staff into communities that were difficult for four-wheeled vehicles to access. After a few months, he was then recruited to work alongside an official Ebola burial team. These teams were established to collect the bodies of all those who died during the epidemic—regardless of the cause of death—and to perform burials safely so as to alleviate one of the primary causes of community Ebola transmission. Each burial team consisted of twelve members: stretcher-bearers, drivers, chlorine sprayers, and navigators. They operated two pristine white vans, one for the team members and the other for the deceased.

Peter's job, which he performed with another bike rider, Alimamy, was to transport two team members who would follow behind the burial team. One of the team members was responsible for taking saliva samples from deceased individuals who were being collected for burial. These samples would later be transported to a lab for processing, which would normally take forty-eight hours. The other staff member a documenter who would fill out a two-page form with information on the deceased and their household. This information was used for contact-tracing purposes and to arrange a quarantine if deemed necessary.

The head of Peter's burial team was an older man, Mr. Kamara, who had previously worked in the Ministry of Health. The rest of the team were young men.

Most had sourced livelihoods prior to the crisis in Freetown's informal economy, working, like Peter, in the transport sector or in small-scale market trading. They by and large welcomed the salaries they were now receiving. The burial team was paid by an international NGO that had assumed management responsibilities from the Ministry of Health for many of the Freetown teams. All team members, including Mr. Kamara, received the equivalent of $100 every Friday morning in an envelope. In addition, the team members were provided with breakfast every morning and with training programs geared toward psychosocial support, which normally included lunch. Peter and his three colleagues, like most responders employed during the epidemic, were paid under the centralized state-operated hazard pay scheme, popularly known as "Ebola money." This entailed a monthly transfer through a phone payment system.

Of course, it was not all rosy. The team was enacting often unpopular new burial regimes that could be both degrading and dangerous (although I was told that no burial team workers in Freetown contracted the disease). Managers sometimes withheld payment to workers, particularly in the hazard pay scheme, or developed informal arrangements in which they would take a percentage of payment in return for the offer of employment.

Peter and his colleagues were, like most people, preoccupied with the shifting horizon that separated Ebola from post-Ebola. They would regularly discuss the latest figures and would speculate, somewhat anxiously, as to what if any benefits they might receive once their rolling contracts were terminated. Many hoped that Ebola jobs would continue after the outbreak. At one point the informal WhatsApp group set up by the team changed its name from "Safe and Dignified Burials" to "Await Post-Ebola Jobs."

I observed the burial team employees rhythmically moving back and forth between pre-Ebola and Ebola positionalities throughout the working day, reflecting the evolving blend of novelties and continuities in their lives and work during the epidemic. In the morning the team members would arrive at their makeshift base on the beach. After breakfast—often rice and beans—the young men would kill time by exercising on the beach, kicking a ball around, comparing updates on phones, texting with friends and sexual partners, and conducting protracted debates on a range of topics. Much of this socialization was typified by a flashy and playful mode of youth masculinity known locally as "bluffing." It was noticeable that as the months of their employment rolled on, team members became better dressed, with new sneakers, leather jackets, large watches, and upgraded phones and electronics. Referring to one of the newly recruited NGO managers who was making money for the first time, Mr. Kamara, the older team manager, who wore the same flat cap and loose brown suit to work every day, once joked to me that "we are existing, even you are existing, but he is *living.* He has two new cars now including a van, and others of them [the administrators] have bought cars too."

After breakfast and time hanging out on the beach, the team would get a call from 117—the service to which all deaths and illnesses, regardless of their Ebola status, were reported—announcing the number of bodies to be collected that day and their location, usually in households or hospital mortuaries. Casual conversations continued in the white vans that the burial teams operated but halted abruptly on arrival at one of the locations for collection. Mr. Kamara or sometimes another team member would communicate with a representative from the mourning family, usually a young man or woman with a smartphone, outlining the arrangements for the burial. Burials took place later the same day before an Ebola test could be processed at a cemetery built for Ebola in the Waterloo district, on the other side of town; this was despite the fact that the majority of deaths were not Ebola-related. Mourners were encouraged to head there as soon as the documenters on the burial team had completed paperwork recording details about the death and the deceased and demographic and contact information for their household. The formal source of this information was the next of kin, but it was typically collected from an educated family member or neighbor. Meanwhile, the stretcher-bearers and chlorine sprayers would be donning the personal protective equipment. This involved adhering to carefully learned safety protocol as well as negotiating with mourning families who were sometimes fazed by these unfamiliar procedures or were resistant to handing over the bodies of their family members.

Weaving between activities was the ongoing evolution and adaptation of working arrangements that emerged around official duties and infrastructures. The work of driving, documenting cases, and taking Ebola swab tests was officially designated for four people, but it could in principle be carried out by one person. Peter and his co–bike rider Alimamy therefore devised ways of covering each other's shifts. Through close observation and informal instruction from the official swab conductor, both learned how to put on and take off the personal protective equipment and conduct the tests safely and efficiently. Peter, an educated university student, could do all the documentation required, while Alimamy, not formally educated, needed assistance. The official documenter had recently taken up secondary employment as a schoolteacher—a job that would probably last longer than this one—and sometimes his cousin came to fill in. The physical resemblance between the two meant that the stand-in could use his cousin's ID card and pass for him. Originally, Peter and Alimamy agreed to trade off, each working one week on and one off. Both owned their own bikes, allowing them to make some money on the side to supplement their formal monthly wages. As a bonus, the person who had worked during the day would collect the daily fuel allowance that was provided for both. This gave Peter and Alimamy additional income; they struck an agreement with the manager at the officially assigned petrol station, according to which they received cash in place of their fuel allocation. The petrol station manager could then resell the petrol, and they fueled their bikes at a cheaper station in the East End.

The universities were reopening, and Peter needed to prepare for exams. He also had additional family commitments; his young daughter, who normally lived with her mother's family in their village upcountry, was staying in town with Peter now. In this and other ways, he was playing a more prominent role in family affairs, made possible by his employment and no doubt necessary by the loss of income among other family members during the crisis. For example, Peter bought a motorbike for his cousin to ride commercially and supported other family members in smaller quotidian ways. Then, without explanation, his pay was cut, probably by a corrupt official at the central hazard pay office. At this point, Alimamy was doing almost all the driving and asked Peter for a weekly payment of 30,000 Le (roughly $5), in addition to Peter's fuel money, reflecting his longer hours. But Peter felt that he was asking for too much and, as a negotiating tool, threatened to use the "legal route." This would entail paying the official documenter—in practice the official documenter's cousin—to cover for him. Meanwhile, Alimamy was still contractually obliged to continue his own job and would be fired if he did not comply. After long and heated negotiations, they settled on an extra payment of 21,000 Le per day, and the working relationship continued.

Underlying the dispute and negotiation between Peter and Alimamy were their attempts to reconcile pre-Ebola commitment, obligations, and aspirations with the conditions in the state of emergency. For Peter, this meant balancing his ongoing studies and commitments to family with the obligations in the Ebola response, solidarities to colleagues, and novel possibilities to benefit from temporary financial flows. When Peter thought that he had finally gained some secure employment and was thinking about his post-Ebola future, his payment was suspended by exploitative officials, undoubtedly aware that many young employees lacked connections or status to reclaim it. Yet, he in turn aimed to use his superior pre-Ebola status as an educated university student over Alimamy who was not educated, by threatening to use the legal route to negotiate a better informal working arrangement between them. This, revealingly, relied on some legally dubious activity. Such acts of reconciling or balancing permeated throughout the activities of the whole team. On a day-to-day basis they were in one moment typical youths, hanging out and playfully bluffing in their fashionable clothes, and in the next moment they were state employees, putting on personal protective equipment and carefully enacting safety procedures that they had been formally trained in.[4]

States of Emergency

Epidemics might be thought of as litmus tests for assessing the capacity of states. National and international responses to emergencies typically entail the (re)-insertion of the state apparatus, or that of other bureaucratic entities, into the lives of ordinary people. Restoring order (at least on paper) requires making legible that which is unknown to the authorities, such as case numbers, the locations of cases, causes of transmission, and economic impact. Legibility and visibilty are key concepts in the analysis of state power. The authority of the state is predicated on its ability to "see" its territory and its subjects and, in a Foucauldian twist, for those subjects to know that they are "seen." In the contemporary world, the state has extended its reach into new domains of knowledge and intervention. This includes, at least in some places, the increasingly centralized management of health and reproductive processes, known as biopolitics. Such knowledge production is put to the test during epidemics when rapid data collection and modeling constitute key aspects of public health responses. The state's ability to know, communicate to, and control its citizens allows for effective regulatory measures to be put in place.

States in the Global South are routinely deemed ill-equipped to respond effectively to emergencies by themselves; international intervention typically goes unquestioned. In a policy document published in August 2014, the World Health Organization wrote that Ebola posed "increasingly serious global health challenges and risks. . . . Clearly a massively scaled and coordinated international response is needed to support affected and at-risk countries in intensifying response activities and strengthening national capacities."[5] The approach that this intervention took was highly bureaucratic, working within, and extending beyond, existing state structures. Populations were made legible in unprecedented ways. Peter and the burial team's work exemplified many aspects of this: the emphasis on Ebola testing and documentation, the state and NGOs taking responsibility for management of the dead, and the centralization of the hazard pay scheme for employing workers.

Massive foreign intervention in Africa should, of course, not go unquestioned. Nor should any state's declaration of a state of emergency. There are questions we should ask. Are inequalities reinforced under the guise of assistance? Are colonial dynamics reproduced? Which people and aspects of their lives are made bureaucratically legible? How are governments and other agencies using emergency powers and do they intend to give them up after the crisis? Critical studies point to the ways that emergencies and interventions are used opportunistically by states, international agencies, and corporations to extend their reach.[6] In the philosopher Georgio Agamben's influential formulation, inspired by Walter Benjamin, the "state of exception" has become the rule in the contemporary world, as state sovereignty is predicated on the ability to override the law rather than enforce it.[7] Some argue that emergencies are themselves artificially constructed in order to further elite interests. This argument is made famous in Naomi Klein's book *The Shock Doctrine*, in which she makes direct connections between "disasters" and the "liberalizing" of new markets, such as after the collapse of the Soviet Union and during the Iraq War.[8] Paul Farmer has elaborated on how global inequalities are reproduced around health emergencies in particular, drawing on his own experience as a doctor on the front lines.[9]

Anthropological research of the Ebola response, particularly in rural settings, reveals how state, military, and international efforts were in large part counterproductive. By the same token, villagers' impressive capacity for adaptation, honed over generations, was routinely disregarded.[10] In some villages in Sierra Leone, customary chiefs initiated and administered their own quarantines. In other villages, secret societies morphed into safe burial teams.[11] And intervening agencies often did not receive reliable information due to villagers' suspicion of the state. It is tempting to apply a similar analysis across the board: communities are always better off by themselves and thus do not want to be made legible by centralized authorities. Acts of resistance during the Ebola emergency have been well documented, representing admirable expressions of agency in the confines of vast inequality.[12]

In Freetown, however, and I suspect in other settings, the story is more layered. Over the decades residents have witnessed a state that is gradually retreating, with economic and political informalization the byproduct of neoliberal "structural adjustment" policies intended to reduce the state's hold on the market. This has had disastrous effects on health systems, which are highly underequipped and underfunded. Experiences of neglect are coupled with experiences of coercion especially for young and marginal workers who routinely face police abuse.[13] Rather than hoping for less "state" in their lives, however, they actually tend to hope for more of it, albeit in a less predatory and more bureaucratic and fair form.[14] While the politics of rebellion from the 1990s have not been forgotten in Sierra Leone, they have seemingly given way to a more conformist ideal in recent times.

The case of commercial bike riders tells this story. The industry took off in the wake of the postwar peace-building intervention, in which young ex-combatants received the capital necessary to buy motorbikes. But the industry has become dogged by exploitative and marginalizing practices, with the BRU featuring ambiguously in the mix. Ebola entailed another major intervention, with new job prospects for young workers. But this time the jobs were actually on the state payroll, with employees becoming official Ebola responders. The

newness and temporariness of the emergency meant that many of the old marginalizing practices featured in state and state-like bureaucracies in Sierra Leone had not yet fully kicked in, which gave it an unusual fairness. Peter and his
colleagues welcomed being incorporated into the state bureaucracy. This was
novel, but it was not alien. Before the outbreak, Peter and Councilor already saw
themselves as quasi bureaucrats, riding between meetings in suits while holding briefcases. But unlike a career in the civil service of old, it was never clear
how long these Ebola jobs would last. Peter and many others responded by striking informal arrangements in order to reconcile their long- and short-term ob-
jectives and responsibilities.

In the end, the success of the official Ebola response was predicated on the abili-
ties of the ordinary workers incorporated into it to make it work. In Freetown,
young employees found much in the response that was in line with their own
ideals, particularly its fairer bureaucratic character and the opportunities it presented for formal employment and official recognition. Being made legible was
not perceived as threatening, as might be expected when considering the critical literature on the topic, but instead was widely welcomed. This makes sense
when considering the coercion and neglect that have characterized informal
workers' experiences of the state in recent decades, which had not yet fully tainted
the novel Ebola bureaucracies, as well as the ways that associations and labor
unions such as the BRU have taken on state-like bureaucratic characteristics together with, somewhat paradoxically, the continuation of rebellious and nonhierarchical discourses and practices.

Work in the Ebola response was not straightforward, however, and adaptations were often deemed necessary. Workers' capacity to operate in both formal
and informal ways was honed through years of experience in operating at the
frontier between the state and the informal economy, in which serious bodily,
legal, and economic risks are ever present, tangled up with the obligations of
family, business, and the law. The Ebola emergency neither introduced nor al-
leviated these problems, but it did allow for new configurations of work and relationships with the state to develop, albeit temporarily.

Human Right did receive the necessary attention and care for his injury to
heal. He stayed close to his family for several months, with Balloon Burst and
other friends visiting him from time to time. The time he spent away from the
streets was somewhat restorative but ultimately unsustainable. He grew restless
being away from the fast life and felt increasingly stuck at home. With his father
unable to earn money due to physical disabilities and his mother's income already overstretched, the pressure for Human Right to find work mounted once

again. A few months after his injury Human Right was riding again. After Ebola, the dangers of commercial bike riding and the tensions between taxi drivers and the state remained, much as they had been before Ebola. Human Right continued to face harassment by the police and suffered other injuries on the road. Balloon Burst found work as a private driver for a well-off family and some years later had his second daughter. While his salary was small, he welcomed the relative security of not needing to hustle on the streets.

HOME TRUTHS

A sick man traveled from his village to stay with relatives in town while he sought treatment. After a week or so, the man passed away. Shortly after, a young woman who had been looking after him fell sick. Her mother rushed her to her father's house, which was a stone's throw away from Foday's home, where I had been staying. She felt that her daughter would be safer away from the gossip and suspicion of their neighbors, who might additionally report them to the authorities. The young woman died at her father's house. This was the first case of Ebola reported in our area. The home was quarantined by the police for twenty-one days, the incubation period for the virus, during which time no one was permitted to enter or leave. Fortunately, no one else in the home became sick or died during this period. Many neighbors doubted whether the young woman had contracted Ebola.

The Ebola emergency presented serious dilemmas for ordinary people caught up in it. In many instances people were forced to decide whether to fulfill important familial obligations and duties to care for the sick and vulnerable—which meant coming close to one another—or follow the official guidance and regulations from the state and international agencies, which tended to emphasize isolating and distancing oneself from others as much as possible.[1] On top of this, with the limited availability of testing (self-administered tests were not available) and the widespread mistrust of state actors, the Ebola status of the sick and the recently deceased often remained undetermined. While it is tempting to consider these kinds of ambiguities and dilemmas as exceptional features of living through epidemic emergencies—and they certainly are exaggerated by such conditions—in

Freetown navigating between contradictory sets of expectations was a rather familiar experience for young people.

This chapter explores the ways that young people in Freetown negotiate between the contrasting yet overlapping social orders of kinship and business in their relationships in and around the home and, more broadly, in their attempts to come of age in a challenging urban environment. Broadly speaking, the social order of kinship is relational, prioritizing obligations to honor and reproduce familial hierarchies as well as participate in the acts of care and material reciprocities that constitute familial relationships. The social order of business is more transactional, speaking to young people's aspirations for independence and self-sufficiency and to social markers of success that draw on both local and global symbols. A great deal of people's social energy before and during the Ebola emergency went into determining which social logic should dominate in a particular instance. Fully separating the two social logics is practically impossible for most youths in urban Africa. To put the paradox simply: you need family to make it in business, and you need business to make it in family. Before we can understand how young people and their families responded to the Ebola epidemic in domestic settings, we must first understand the social dynamics and conflicts that preceded and continued to play out during the emergency.

Quarantining—an epidemiological technique that goes back at least as far as biblical times—was a core element of the official Ebola response. During the outbreak, quarantined homes formed distinctive landmarks in Freetown's residential neighborhoods. A makeshift tape perimeter was staked out around the home. Police officers were stationed outside to protect against leaving and entering. Essential supplies—food, drink, toiletries—and new mattresses, in the case of quarantine after a death, were typically provided by international and state authorities, alongside informal support from neighbors and friends. Demarcating a single home, however, is by no means a straightforward task in many parts of Freetown. Rooms in multiple-family compounds often interlock, and some houses are subdivided into smaller family units. Demarcating a household is an even trickier task, given the flexibility of residential patterns. The occupants in the homes that I lived in changed regularly, with extended family and friends staying for days, months, or years at a time. I heard of some cases in which visitors who were stopping by the home were forced to undergo quarantine with the rest of the household due to being with them at time of the arrival of the police.

When I spoke to those who had gone through quarantine, their responses were rather mixed. Some complained that neighbors had distanced themselves, declining support during their time of need. Sometimes they invoked the NGO-inspired language of "stigmatization" when making such claims. Taking it even further, I heard several stories of quarantines being issued after neighbors had deceptively reported on other neighbors through the 117 emergency service while in a dispute or argument. It was as if quarantine had joined the established arsenal of familial pressure, the police, courts, and witchcraft as weapons for conducting neighborly conflict. I heard about other cases in which quarantines were actively welcomed—or even self-imposed—as a means of receiving coveted supplies from the authorities.

The home was in many ways the front line of the epidemic, a fact that was well recognized by public authorities and ordinary people. Home-based care, such as looking after the sick and preparing a corpse for burial, was a primary cause of viral transmission.[2] Even in normal circumstances, home-based care is prevalent in Freetown even in cases of severe illness, given how drastically underresourced hospitals and clinics are, along with prohibitive costs for treatment. Many of the bylaws and epidemiological measures employed during the Ebola state of emergency—such as lockdowns, curfews, and community monitoring—directly targeted the home and families even where there were no suspected Ebola cases.

The home during Ebola was a notably ambiguous space. The economic fallout experienced during the crisis made many people heavily reliant on those closest by. Some were forced to spend more time at home than they were used to if, for example, they did not have money to spend. Regulations on movement and lockdowns also forced people to stay at home. The home could be a site of refuge and sustenance during these hard times and yet also one of boredom and shame. I remember Alhassan, Foday's older brother, who normally enjoyed visiting friends and girlfriends around town, complaining to me that "Ebola is like being stuck in the compound all day—it is boring."[3] The home could also be a site of physical danger. The virus was transmitted via contact with bodily fluids, which typically took place between intimate and proximate relations. Harboring a sick relative ran the risk of not only catching the virus but also severe legal penalties.

In global health and international development discourse, these kinds of challenges are often framed around the concept of stigmatization. Stigmatization is a serious issue, entering public awareness partly as a response to the horrific prejudice faced by those living with HIV/AIDS, often from already marginalized communities across the globe. Stigmatization of Ebola victims during the 2014–2016 epidemic spawned a number of high-profile initiatives to combat it on the ground. However, the mixed responses to quarantine reported to me—as well as my firsthand experiences of lockdown, detailed in chapter 4—paint a more varied and nuanced picture of the home in crisis. Stigmatization is only one dimension of ambiguous social dynamics that far exceed the contours of health and risk in a conventional biomedical sense.[4] Understanding this dynamic requires an analysis that takes into account the quality of social relations in both normal times and times of emergency. It also requires careful attention both to what is verbalized and what goes unspoken. As will be described here, ambiguity and marginalization in the home was not introduced by Ebola but instead preceded it. However, during Ebola young people gained unusual clarity on old problems that they faced around care and coming of age.

This insight has major implications for our understandings of the relationship between emergency and the home and compels a rethinking of tacit assumptions that domestic space, or the private sphere, is essentially orderly and safe, only becoming disordered and dangerous in exceptional circumstances. This is a deep-rooted staple of Western thought, although it might be better understood as a deeply held fantasy. Wherever you go around the world and even in the world of mythology and story, the home is the stage for both care and conflict, almost as two sides of the same coin. For young people in Freetown, conflict around the home centered on disputes concerning the appropriate expectations and relations classifications of different fundamental social orders in which they were simultaneously enmeshed, which I here call the orders of "kinship" and "business."

Ambiguous Houses

It did not take me long to taste the various flavors of ambiguity within the homes that I stayed in and frequented in Freetown. I was regularly reminded of how just below the surface of seemingly convivial and close relationships lurked long-harbored tensions. I was struck by people's generosity and care and the willingness for poor households to accept new residents. At the same time, though, I learned that such gestures were sometimes interpreted as harmful and exploitative. Just as strangers could become kin through living together, so too could kin become strangers and forced out of the home. The dependence that many of my neighbors had on those living around them was seen as both a source of strength and a source of vulnerability, with trust and reliance often morphing into secrecy and suspicion.

In Freetown, the home was a particularly ambivalent space for young men and women. Even before the epidemic, young people I became close to would spend much of the day in and around the house.[5] Many did not have regular jobs to go to or money to spend. In the absence of formal employment, it was often around the home and the neighborhood that business did happen. Opportunities for informal work might come up, or there were the ongoing circulations of money and things to attend to. Being indebted to friends, family, and neighbors was commonplace, and repaying creditors often required pressuring your own debtors to square up, so things would often get messy. Channels of opportunity and sustenance in the home could easily flip into exploitation and indebtedness, reenforcing dependencies and threatening the real dangers of social stagnation and decline. Home ownership, however unobtainable, remains a primary marker of social adulthood, and hanging around the family home can be interpreted as a sign of laziness and immaturity.[6] These value systems are legacies from an earlier era when wage labor in factories, on docks, and on the state payroll were realistic possibilities for young people in Freetown, as well as harkening to kinship-based systems of land tenure, which are more prominent in rural areas.

Ambiguity around the home is readily observable in Freetown simply from the terms that family members, neighbors, and friends use to greet one another. One set of terms is clearly derived from the language of family: "bro," "sister," "auntie," "uncle," "pa," "ma," and so on. These are applied much more widely than among formal kin. Another set of common terms is derived from the language of business and work, and yet these terms are used regularly in and around the home and neighborhood. These include "senior man," "boss-man," "*grand-jon*" (male boss), "*sisi*" (female boss), "manager," and "*bor bor*" (apprentice). The rule is generally to acknowledge seniority by using appropriate terms, although sometimes this rule is jokingly inverted. Sometimes relative seniority between two people is itself ambiguous or circumstantially dependent, so different terms might be used at different times.

Greeting is not an incidental formality in Freetown but instead is an essential part of community life. It was through learning how to greet others appropriately—after quite a few slipups—that I also learned where the boundaries of my neighborhood community really were. If I was walking along the major road feeding into the neighborhood, passerby did not normally greet or expect to be greeted. As soon as I turned into the side street or path, I was told off if I did not greet a passerby appropriately, especially if the person was senior to me.

The coexistence and interchangeability of terms of greeting that derive from the orders of kinship and business, while in themselves serving to demarcate social relationships, point to instabilities and ambiguities between these different social orders.[7] The inclination to view a relationship alternately through either lens produces two distinct visions of the expectations involved, which youths are particularly prone to getting caught between. A great deal of social energy goes into determining which social order's perspective should take precedent in any given circumstance. An everyday example is a young person doing household chores. Examined through the lens of kinship, this looks like the fulfillment of a familial obligation. Seen through the lens of business, it could easily be interpreted as exploitative, unpaid labor.

In the sections that follow, I describe episodes from three different domestic settings I knew well in the Congo Town neighborhood that serve to illustrate the patterns of ambiguity, conflict, and resolution that characterized life in and around the home. The first case is in Foday's room and parlor, a small two-room house in which several young men lived together, including myself for the first half of a long period of fieldwork between 2013 and 2015. The second is in the Bangura family compound where I lived for the second half of this period composed of several closely connected family units. And the third is on the Cole land, adjacent to the family compound, where there was a dispute between an uncle and a nephew. All three cases preceded and spanned the Ebola epidemic, in part revealing the ways that experiences of and responses to the emergency were entangled with ongoing relational dynamics.

Foday's Room and Parlor

Foday, my first host, the young taxi driver and musician we met in chapter 1, lived in a small house located near to the base of the valley around which the Congo Town neighborhood lay. The external walls were built with cement blocks, and the internal walls were makeshift medium-density fiberboard. The roof was made of corrugated metal sheets. The house was not connected to running water; we filled buckets from a nearby tap. Access to the house was via a steep rocky path down from the main road. Foday, in his midtwenties, built the home on land belonging to the fourth and only surviving wife of Molay, his deceased grandfather who was the patriarch of the family and had migrated to Freetown in the 1950s. Foday held a leasehold agreement, according to which the property, including the structure that Foday built, would return to his grandfather's wife after six years unless he then paid rent to her.

As noted earlier, I had gotten to know Foday during a previous visit to Freetown. He agreed to host me when I arrived. Life in the home was fun and stimulating, but it was also ultimately a place I found challenging to live in. Many youths from the neighborhood would hang out there, playing video games, watching DVDs of TV shows and movies, or listening to and recording music. The atmosphere was often playful and quite male. This was somewhat balanced by the neighbors' place, which housed mostly female residents under a strong maternal figure. The proximity between the homes, both physical and social, made it feel at times like we were all living together under one roof.

When Foday was not driving a taxi, he focused on music. He ran a small recording studio—located in the front room—that would typically operate at night when electricity was more reliable than in the day, when there were regular power cuts. The normal sleeping arrangements were me sharing the bed with Foday, with Umaru and Sam, two of Foday's male cousins, sleeping in the parlor on the sofa and a makeshift mattress when recording had stopped. Umaru was slightly older than Foday, as the lines on his forehead revealed. He was a teenager during the civil war, when he fought as a rebel soldier, although he did not talk about this much. Umaru was now a comedian by profession and carried a warm and playful disposition through much of his social life. He presented a weekly comedy radio program and was hired by people in the area to perform at parties, but this work had not yet translated into significant financial reward. Umaru and Foday had a very intimate friendship, which they described as "brotherhood." Sam, a few years younger than Foday, was the *bor bor* of the house who had come to stay with Foday after Sam's father died. Sam was young but ambitious about progressing in life. Foday's father had asked him to take Sam under his wing as a driving apprentice, and he agreed.

While all three were cousins and roughly the same age, their reasons for living together and the character of their relationships went beyond family. Foday had hundreds of cousins, but Umaru and Foday had met at the funeral of an elder within the family, and their relationship soon became close-knit. They became collaborators in the shared project of gaining traction in Freetown's entertainment scene. Their friendship also involved daily acts of tactile playfulness, sharing clothes and food, and attending church and family events together.

Sam and Foday's relationship was initiated by Foday's father but took on a life of its own. Sam expected Foday to become his "boss" and "big brother" and to initiate him into the driving business by teaching him how to drive and then employing him as a driver. From Sam's perspective, becoming close to Foday and working around the house was a way of encouraging Foday to take him under his wing and give him the tools to earn a living. On a day-to-day basis, Sam performed household tasks such as cleaning the house, washing clothes, and collecting items from the shops. Foday sometimes gave Sam portions of food, which Sam often received from family and neighbors, and provided him with a floor to sleep on. This was a common arrangement for young people moving into a household; a roof over their head was conditional on either contributing money (if they had an external income) or working for the house.

The three relationships, while built around acts of care, mutual support, and intimate proximity, were ultimately unstable. Umaru and Foday's relationship became increasingly strained. While Umaru, as a more senior and well-connected person in the entertainment business, was in many ways a desirable partner for Foday, Umaru soon began to look like something of a liability; Foday was putting more into relationship on a day-to-day basis. The difficulties were compounded when Umaru, while using a motorbike that Foday had obtained (in exchange for his car), left the keys in the ignition at the top of the path leading down to the house while he ran down to fetch something. When he reached the top of the path again, the motorbike was gone. This incident, however, appeared to me to reveal—rather than necessarily cause—a dysfunctionality in Foday and Umaru's relationship. Umaru came with his mother to the house to officially beg for Foday's forgiveness, as they did not have the money to replace the bike, and Foday reluctantly accepted. He admitted to me afterward that he did not feel that he had much of a choice.

The relationship between Sam and Foday became even more riddled with resentments and animosity. Foday never got around to teaching Sam to drive, which was Sam's primary goal in living with Foday. Lessons were still held up as a possibility by Foday whenever Sam brought up the subject but were continually delayed when it came to practicalities. Increasingly Sam felt that he was being exploited and that his junior status of *bor bor* was becoming further cemented. Sam once said to me with reference to Foday that "we should be working together as brothers, so we can develop, but he doesn't take other people's problem seriously."

These grievances were rarely expressed directly, however. If they were, then they would provide the concrete evidence necessary for aggrieved parties to formally complain to higher authorities, such as Foday's father in this case. Or they might, people feared, lead to indirect retaliations, such as sharing negative stories about each other with others in the neighborhood or family or through witchcraft attacks.[8] Rather, grievances were enacted symbolically around the house, a stage on which expectations were renegotiated on a daily basis. Sam stopped helping out so much in the house, and Foday started doing much more of his own cleaning. Equally, Sam would accept Foday's offers of food much less regularly, finding food instead among other neighbors and friends with whom he had close relationships, independent of Foday.

On one occasion Foday, Umaru, and I were sharing a plate of rice and cassava leaf stew with fish prepared by one of our neighbors. Foday called out to Sam, who was sitting on the veranda listening to music in his headphones, "Come, let's eat." After a few loud shouts and no response from Sam, Foday, frustrated, exclaimed, "He does this too much! This is the last time that I am going to offer him food." For Sam, these gestures demonstrated that he was not entirely reliant on Foday. For Foday, they signified that he owed Sam less. Eventually Sam started spending nights elsewhere, although he left his clothes at Foday's as a marker that he still had a place there. In one tense moment, Foday moved Sam's clothes from their usual spot when he was cleaning the house one weekend, sending the signal that Sam was no longer welcome in his home. Eventually after three years together, Sam moved out to stay with a friend elsewhere in a more equal-footed relationship, similar to that between Umaru and Foday.

But Sam was obsessed with finding a place of his own. He told me once, with a tone that conveyed frustration mixed with quiet resolve, that "if I move out, I believe I will be able to progress more if I am on my own." He attempted to negotiate with the same grandma in the family who owned Foday's land to build on a small plot of land nearby, but this proved challenging given Sam's relatively distant connection to the main family compound in the area (where none of his nuclear family lived). It was notable to me that Sam seemed to see having his own place as a means to an end, a way of getting on in life more generally, rather than an end in itself. The lack of a place of his own was not the consequence of having no regular, good employment, but, as he described it, was instead almost the reason for it. The logic became clear when Sam explained to me that "Foday would respect Umaru more if he had his own place. At his level, he should have his own place." This exemplified a paradox that was central for many young people such as Sam and Umaru. Getting on required at one and the same time living under the protection of close support figures, who straddled the boundaries between kinship and business, and being independent from them.

The Bangura Family Compound

After eight months or so with Foday, I transferred to a small room and parlor of my own within a family compound only a few hundred meters up the hill from where Foday lived. It was shortly after this move that Ebola regulations began coming into effect. My move was partly in response to tensions in Foday's home, which felt exacerbated by my presence in the already crowded space that also contributed to some tension between Foday and myself. Perhaps this move was part of my own coming of age in Freetown. The family compound belonged to the Bangura family. I was particularly close to James, the oldest son in the Bangura family, who was friends with Foday, although their relationship too was rocky. In the main house in the compound, which comprised three small bedrooms, a bathroom, a living room, and a veranda, lived James's father Jonathan—who grew increasingly frail during the course of my fieldwork—and his four children. Jonathan's wife Leah also lived in the home with her three children. Leah was a regular churchgoer in her late forties and a strong maternal presence in the compound. In adjacent homes lived several other relatives, including James's uncle and aunt and their daughters and his great-uncle. During my stay several occupants came and went, giving the extended household a shifting character.

The social structure of the home was fairly typical of Freetown family compounds. Unlike Foday's room and parlor, the Bangura home was intergenerational. However, while hierarchies defined by formal notions of kinship were acknowledged in principle, in practice roles and responsibilities were also continually renegotiated. Jonathan, a cook by profession, was designated as head of the compound. Strictly speaking, the most senior family member was Mohammed, a short, loudly spoken builder, nicknamed "Boys" because he was often found with an entourage of young apprentices. Mohammed was a son of the *mami* (senior woman) who founded the compound. The mami had arrived from upcountry in the 1950s and acquired the land, initially to establish a women's initiation society. This still operated during my fieldwork though in a much less prominent form; there was one dark room in the corner of the compound to which only the initiated had access. Mohammed had never married, had not been educated, and did not hold a steady job or have a steady income. His precarity was undoubtedly exacerbated by a heavy drinking habit and somewhat erratic behavior. He had several children, but many of them were estranged from him. As a result, his seniority within the family was significantly depleted.

Jonathan was frail during my time at the compound, and he died shortly after I left. His wife Leah had taken over some of his professional responsibilities as a cook and had also taken over many of the key decision-making processes in the household, another mark of seniority. James, a cook and waiter, also became more involved in managing the house at this stage. He took over as head of the household alongside Leah when his father passed away. Uncle Samuel, a distant relative who lacked any claim to the land, did not attempt to replace Jonathan as head of the household but, as an educated and respected schoolteacher, held seniority and respect within the compound, which was regularly acknowledged at family gatherings.

Beyond the more formalized decision-making processes—such as at family events and gatherings—hierarchies within the home were performed on a day-to-day basis through various enactments of a "chain of command." For example, senior people were entitled to and would regularly send junior people to the shops to buy something for themselves or for the house. This activity could only be performed this way; sending a more senior person would be seen as highly insulting. For people who were closely positioned in terms of status, sending each other was a semi-humorous way of asserting seniority.

Another example involved the distribution of the daily pot of rice and *plasas* (sauces/soups) that were cooked in the home. The more senior people in the home would have their own portions set aside, often with larger quantities of meat or fish. Once they had finished eating, it was their responsibility to redistribute portions of food to the more junior members of the household. Food sharing would often extend beyond the established residents of the home, serving to nourish broader networks of relatedness and establish their connection to the home. As one friend put it, "Your base is where you eat." The passing down of food could reassert hierarchies, but food could also be shared in more humbling ways.

Zainab was a long-term resident of the compound, a young woman I came to know as James's sister. I discovered much later that she was not formally related to the Bangura family. She was the longtime long-distance girlfriend of James's first cousin Victor, whom James had grown up with in their native village. James was particularly close to her as a result. Victor had been living in Ghana for several years, where he was training to become a Catholic priest, which created some ambiguity about the status of his relationship with Zainab. There were expectations of celibacy, of course, but Victor did not seem intent on adhering to this religiously.

Zainab slept in a room that she rented immediately adjacent to the main family rooms. She often did her cooking separately, which gave her a degree of independence. She was studying and was also working at a hotel in town as a receptionist. At one point she juggled two full-time jobs at separate hotels. She had incorporated herself into the family—beyond her relatively fragile connection through James's cousin—partly by contributing to family expenses. She made especially generous contributions to family programs such as weddings but also contributed by being a respected and caring figure in the compound. For much of the time that I was living there, Zainab took care of two children from the Bangura family whose mother had unexpectedly passed away until they were transferred to a more permanent residence. These activities strengthened her position within the family, and she was regularly called to family meetings where important decisions were made. However, her connection to the family was never entirely stable. In the physical absence of her boyfriend, she kept local boyfriends without letting it be widely known; this was a common practice but nevertheless was somewhat looked down on. These relationships involved not only companionship but also some additional income from which the family benefitted. At the same time, though, Zainab's other relationships could be used against her when asserting her claims to the residence.

Not everyone coming into the household did so with such success and acceptance as Zainab. For a few rocky months Leah's niece Kadiatu, a young woman in her mid to late twenties, came to live with us. Kadiatu enjoyed an active social life. Leah had taken Kadiatu under her wing; Kadiatu's mother, Leah's younger sister, did not have the resources to look after her. In addition, Kadiatu had four children fathered by various partners and was unable to look after them. Leah explained to me that she hoped the compound would provide Kadiatu with a stable environment until she was able to settle down herself. A condition, presumably unspoken, of Kadiatu living in the compound was that she would contribute to daily household tasks such as cooking and cleaning.

While Kadiatu's kinship connection to the house was more direct than Zainab's and Kadiatu was older, her lack of external income (she had neither a job nor financially supportive partners) made her manifestly lower status within the home. She was tasked with household work alongside the children and teenagers in the house, one of whom she was sharing a bed with. Before Kadiatu's pregnancies, Leah had previously been sponsoring her education. Kadiatu expected Leah to pay for her to continue her education now that she was living under her or to take a course such as in cookery. But Kadiatu saw this as a false promise that was dangled like a carrot on a stick while she cooked and cleaned, not unlike Foday's promise to teach his younger cousin Sam to drive.

Tension progressively grew in Kadiatu and Leah's relationship, coming to a head over several issues. The first was Kadiatu's habit of leaving the home in evenings, sometimes coming back very late or spending the night elsewhere. Kadiatu had recently started seeing Umaru, Foday's cousin, and would sometimes spend the night with him on the floor of his parlor, where I had been previously living. Leah worried about Kadiatu. Some nights she sat on the chair on the veranda waiting for her niece to come home. The second issue was business-related. Leah had loaned Kadiatu money to start a small fish-selling enterprise. The plan was to buy from a local fisherman and then sell the fish door to door. What happened instead, according to Leah's plausible reports, was that Kadiatu borrowed fish from market traders downtown on credit and sold them on without significant profit while "eating" (wastefully spending) most of Leah's seed money. She was slowly repaying Leah's loan until she found herself in debt over her head to the fish seller downtown. Leah reluctantly forked out more cash to bail Kadiatu out.

Part of the problem was the ambiguity in Leah and Kadiatu's relationship. Leah regarded Kadiatu as her daughter while she was living in her house. But Kadiatu did not regard Leah as her mother and thus did not feel that she needed to obey house rules, such as coming home early and working around the house. Perhaps she saw Leah more as an investor. During one heated argument that took place outside the house, Leah cried, "If your child does not act correctly, you will feel it," a statement that got straight to the heart of the matter. When Kadiatu came close to Leah she became both a family member and a business partner. But the business project, while perhaps being a source of connection early on, had ultimately strained their familial bond. Finally Kadiatu left the house, leaving her tensions with Leah alive and unresolved.

After many months of bubbling tension, Kadiatu came to beg Leah. This was an official way of talking grievances out and apologizing. The meeting was formally witnessed by several neighbors and significant family members and was chaired by the young formally dressed pastor of the Pentecostal church that James, Umaru, Kadiatu, and Foday attended. During the course of the meeting, grievances were openly expressed. The pastor talked about how this was an opportunity to "start again." At one point he told Leah, "You are in fact the mother, this is your child," thus clarifying the underlying tension as well as astutely drawing direct attention to the root cause of the problems. Leah was still as she heard this, her eyes slowly welling up. It was only through confronting this issue that their tension could resolve, although it seemed to take Kadiatu's moving out of the home to get there. As the event reached its climax, Kadiatu, in line with tradition yet with a hint of knowing exaggeration, fell to her knees, touched Leah's feet, and begged for forgiveness. Both women looked each other in the eyes and started laughing.

The Cole Land

The land adjacent to the Bangura compound was owned by Mr. Cole, an elder who had returned upcountry to his native village. When Mr. Cole passed away, the land became the object of dispute between his son, Brima, and his brother, Andrew, both of whom resided there. I had become friendly with Brima, who was close to both James Bangura and Foday, acting like something of a big brother to them as they were growing up. Brima was in his early to midthirties. He worked as the intelligence officer at the local police station, which was a steady job, but he was badly and unreliably paid. Brima was a well-known figure in the neighborhood. He would act as an informal consultant for residents when they were considering taking an issue through the formal legal system. Brima lived in a small room and parlor with his wife Sally and their two young children.

The Cole land was subdivided into several units containing smaller homes like Brima and Sally's. By the road was a much larger multistory compound that had been built by his uncle Andrew—a former police officer—and Andrew's wife Fatu. Andrew had made a significant amount of money when he was posted at the airport, having become embroiled in the illegal cocaine trade. The operation was eventually busted. Andrew was scapegoated by the police force and was dismissed from his duties and sent to prison for some time. Now out of prison, he had become an established member of the community and the family. Andrew lived primarily off rent collected from the houses on the family land as well as from a small grocery store that Fatu ran from the ground floor of their house. Brima, however, was permitted to collect rent from the group of houses directly next to his own, which supplemented his own salary from the police force.

Mr. Cole's death threw these arrangements up in the air. The documents for the land were in his name and in his possession. According to Brima, his father had intended to hand over the documents to him as his wife's oldest son (although he also had children with other partners) but had never gotten around to putting Brima's name on the documents. Nonetheless, Brima would have had strong claim to the property if he was able to access the original documents. In a cruel twist of fate, his father's corpse had been rapidly collected by an official Ebola burial team—according to state of emergency protocols—while Brima was still on the road. And the documents for the land were in his father's pocket! Brima's account, regardless of its veracity, speaks volumes about the ways that the tensions of the Ebola emergency animated existing family dynamics.

Andrew, as Mr. Cole's younger brother, was a senior member of the family and a longtime resident on the land and had a strong claim to it after his brother's passing. Such disputes between children and siblings of the deceased are commonplace in claims to land in Sierra Leone, given ambiguities in inheritance protocols. The conflict blew up when Andrew began collecting rent from the whole property, ignoring the previous arrangement in which Brima received a share of the rental income. Brima felt that was under increasing pressure to leave the property. He saw his half-brother Alfred, who shared the same father, being groomed by Andrew to replace Brima as the property's caretaker. But Brima bitterly interpreted this as the same ultimately manipulative form of care that he too had received from Andrew.

Andrew had helped bring Brima into the police force and, in a more amorphous sense, into adulthood. As Brima put it, he "gave me my first Guinness stout" (a popular bottled beer). Brima's indebtedness to and respect for his uncle were interwoven with feelings of betrayal and resentment. All of this was crystallized for Brima when Andrew spoke to him at Mr. Cole's funeral. Brima told me that "I distinctly remember him saying, 'I will look after you now.' It was an ironical statement." The event of death brought to the fore competing interests that had been suppressed beneath the convivial surface of everyday life shared by neighbors in a close-knit social environment. Brima had taken on a nurturing role with Andrew and Fatu's daughters, regularly helping them with their schoolwork and giving them lunch money. Likewise, Brima and his wife Sally's daughter, Aisha, went regularly to Andrew and Fatu's to play and eat.

For Brima, the conflict was a test of pride, dignity, and resolve. Andrew and Fatu "did not have mind" to tell him directly to leave. Instead, they employed indirect means to make it intolerable for Brima to stay, thereby forcing him and his family to depart by their own volition. This approach, I was told, was "the typical African way." Brima was convinced that Andrew and Fatu wanted to prove that he could not survive without collecting rent from the property:

"They wanted to see me suffer." Brima believed that they had intentionally cut off his electricity by contacting someone from the National Power Authority through another neighbor who worked there and had similarly distanced himself from Brima. Brima was also sure that Fatu was targeting him and his family through occult rituals. He accused Fatu of preparing a spiritually poisoned salad for him to eat. However, as with his electricity being intentionally cut off, this was indirect and difficult to confirm.

Brima isolated himself for some time, not socializing with his neighbors as he normally would have done. He started building a small house on the outskirts of town, where he had bought land a while back and had been planning to build. He did not intend to give up the fight by leaving, but the knowledge that there was to be a place where his family could "live in peace" and "keep things to themselves" was a source of comfort to him. It also proved that he could survive without collecting the rent. Brima was clearly insecure about being seen as overly dependent on others for a helping hand.

The instability of Brima's emotional state during this period seemed to me to correspond closely to the progress on his new house. Each stage that was completed gave Brima more confidence, marking the transition from being socially reclusive and cut off to engaged in the community. The relationships he had cultivated with Andrew's daughters were also key in overcoming the hostilities. Andrew's oldest daughter came to Brima's house to appeal him to become close again with her family, claiming that they were acting stubbornly because they had consumed poisoned food prepared by Andrew's former wife, which had "changed their minds." Brima remained cautious about letting down his guard and reconnecting. "Trust takes a long time to build back," he told me, not least because he feared that exposing himself further to them would enable them to take advantage of him again. He suspected that Fatu's call to perform a *sara* (ceremony) with his daughter Aisha after she was ill so as to protect her from witchcraft was in fact a means of spiritually attacking her and them, of coming close with bad intentions. In turn, Brima felt aggrieved that the close and supportive relationship he had built with Andrew and Fatu's daughters had not been acknowledged.

As a form of cease-fire, Brima and Sally went to beg formally to Andrew and Fatu in the presence of Mr. Barrie, a respected community elder and a prominent member of the local mosque. Mr. Barrie acknowledged the "big *wahala*" that everyone was talking about, gently shaking his head as he spoke with a tone of quiet but dignified authority. Although Brima believed that he was in the right, as the less senior person it was his responsibility to apologize to his uncle. Andrew was visibly upset about bad language that Brima had used against him and, in a Shakespearean turn, had claimed that Brima had actively spread the rumor around the family that Andrew had killed Brima's father. The session was an opportunity for Brima to voice his grievances against his uncle, and some measure of peace was achieved. The issue over ownership of the compound was not resolved, and Andrew continued to collect all the rent, but the "bad feeling in the heart" was ameliorated. Shortly afterward, Brima told me that "dignity is more important than money."

For Brima, a key moment in the reconciliation process was the eventual celebration of his and Sally's wedding anniversary after some delay. The big sound system blasting out the latest Nigerian Afrobeat music was a proud message to Andrew and Fatu that he was living his life to the fullest rather than suffering. He sent them and his other neighbors food and drinks from the party. It did not seem coincidental that it was during this semipublic celebration that Brima and Fatu finally spoke at length in the middle of the dancing area, visibly—although not audibly—airing what they had been holding inside.

Conflicts of Care

The three cases outlined above all speak to conflicts of care within and around the home, despite significant differences in living arrangements and domestic structures. Ambiguity between different sets of expectations around care and domestic roles seems to bubble below the surface, erupting in moments of dispute, and then sinks back down when things are, at least temporarily, resolved. Care itself has a double-edged quality. In one moment it is experienced as nourishing and supportive, and in the next, particularly for young people, it is infantilizing and exploitative.

Such conflicting attributes of care get to the core of the almost inevitably unstable dynamics of human intimacy. In Sierra Leone, there are well-developed ways of thinking and talking about the tensions of home-based care. As elsewhere, witchcraft is understood as a malevolent force transmitted by those close by through the sharing of food or the targeting of victims in their sleep. For example, in the Cole land dispute, Brima accused his aunt of poisoning a salad that she had prepared for him. The discourse of witchcraft speaks to the kinds of day-to-day ambiguities and conflicts that I have described in this chapter. For youths in Freetown, care around the home can be stigmatizing and deadly—socially, economically, and emotionally—just as it is nourishing and vital.

As discussed in chapter 1, the dual potential for freedom and slavery engendered in kinship goes back at least as far as the Atlantic slave trade. But in twenty-first-century Freetown, it finds particular expression through the demands of kinship and business that are simultaneously placed on domestic and familial relationships. The fulfillment of young people's desires to become somebody typically requires acceptance within familial networks at the same time as it requires some degree of independent economic worth through land, home ownership or an income. In practice, however, both parts of the puzzle are dynamically—and often paradoxically—interconnected: you need family to make it in business, and business to make it in family. Young people find themselves wanting recognition within the home and then wanting to leave altogether.

In the room and parlor, Foday and Sam were cousins and so in kinship terms were roughly on an even footing. In business terms, Foday was Sam's boss even though the promised driving apprenticeship never materialized. This relegated Sam to a junior role in the home, which came with a heavy load of household chores. When Sam became increasingly dissatisfied with the lack of progress on the business front and the chores, he attempted to renegotiate his place in the home by demonstrating that he could survive independently. This was symbolized by rejecting Foday's invitation to eat from his plate. In another circumstance, Foday's invitation would be read as a caring and generous gesture. But in this instance, it was interpreted by Sam as a cruel act of manipulation.

There were similar patterns in the Bangura family compound. Although Zainab's formal connection to the family was weak because she had not married in, she had successfully become kin by contributing to household and family projects, funded in part by income that she drew in externally from her employment as a hotel receptionist. Kadiatu's story was the reverse. Work in the house felt exploitative and demeaning, and her failed business enterprise with Leah, her aunt, resulted in their relationship being suspended. When their relationship was finally reconciled, it was possible only by the reinforcement of Kadiatu's subservient position to Leah.

Finally, in the Cole land dispute, competing claims between an uncle, Andrew, and a nephew, Brima, became interlaced with other measures of seniority, notably professional and economic. Andrew had helped to bring Brima into the police force, thus playing a large role in his development. But after his father had died, Brima had found his uncle's promise to look after him threatening because he feared that it would now stunt his development, restricting his independence. In the end, however, Brima decided to not leave the compound even if it meant accepting his uncle's seniority.

These patterns, or cycles, within caring relationship around the home were characterized by prolonged phases of ambiguity, punctuated by moments of clarity, typically when tensions reached the boiling point. This is not dissimilar from Victor Turner's classic notion of a social drama: "a limited area of transparency on the otherwise opaque surface of regular, uneventful social life."[9] It was during these moments of domestic crisis, or emergency, that the entangled yet conflicting modalities of care—supportive and exploitative—and the primary registers of status—kinship and business—unraveled, with participants being able to clearly glimpse their constituent parts.

It is not coincidental that these events and the discussions that I had with participants during and around them were critical in developing my own understanding of the foundational social dynamics of the home. And yet, nonverbal gestures were often just as significant if not more so in making sense of and ultimately resolving tensions than what was spoken: Sam's refusal to eat from Foday's plate, Kadiatu touching Leah's feet, and Brima and Fatu's exchange on the dance floor.[10] The interplay between different ways of knowing—spoken or unspoken and embodied—that come to fore in an emergency, whether micro, such as family dramas, or macro, most obviously during the time of Ebola, is a theme that will crop up again in the chapters to come.

This chapter began with a discussion of Ebola quarantines and the mixed responses they elicited. In some cases, people complained about being cut off from their established networks of care. In other cases, being cut off was understood as the latest development in an ongoing tussle between residents or neighbors, quite separate to the Ebola epidemic. And some Freetown residents sought out quarantines because of the material benefits that came with them.

It was well known that Ebola spread through channels of intimacy and familial care; much of the public health messaging directly spoke to this. Ebola was cruel because it rendered care for the sick and the dead potentially life-threatening for the caregiver. Alternatively, falling ill could lead to the sick being stigmatized, with normal expectations of care morphing into exclusion. But contact, sharing, and care among networks of family and friends was crucial in getting through the emergency and maintaining important social relationships. Thus, Freetown residents faced major dilemmas in adhering to the demands of the official Ebola response, which tended to emphasize separation and distancing oneself from others, and the demands of family and friends to come close to one another during a crisis.

How new was all of this? This chapter has suggested that at their core, such ambiguities around intimate and domestic relationships were far from novel in Freetown. In fact, young people in Freetown prior to the Ebola epidemic were greatly preoccupied with navigating between different social orders and negotiating their contradictory sets of expectations. In the domestic spaces of the home and the neighborhood—settings that are central for African youths but widely overlooked—the dominant social orders are those of kinship and business. As we have seen, determining which social logic should take precedent in a particular instance is foundational to the disputes and resolutions outlined in this chapter. The fundamental mutual interdependence and yet irreconcilability of the two logics, underpinned by a broader economic context of material scarcity and extraction, is a central factor in the current manifestation of what has been called the crisis of youth in Africa.

But the Ebola emergency did represent a new vantage point regarding an old problem. The disease was an alarmingly physical and exaggeratedly cruel manifestation of conflicts of care around the home. Ebola revealed new dimensions of long-standing social ambiguities and came with new ways of talking about and responding to them. Sometimes this amounted to unusual clarity and novel solutions to ongoing and deep-rooted challenges. While domestic and intimate relationships significantly shaped young people's experiences of the emergency, the emergency in turn reanimated and reconfigured established ordinary social processes. These themes are developed further in chapter 4 and chapter 5, which center in part on developments in the Bangura family during Ebola.

EXTRAORDINARY ORDINARY

Before the first day of a three-day lockdown in Freetown, Sierra Leone president Ernest Bai Koroma gave the following speech:

> Everybody in every house in every community in this country is very important in our fight against Ebola. Avoid touching each other, avoid eating bush meat, avoid visiting the sick, avoid attending funerals, report illnesses and deaths to the nearest health facility or call 117. We know some of the things we are asking you to do are difficult. But life is better than these difficulties. Today the life of everyone is at stake, but we will get over this difficulty if all do what we have been asked to do. Ebola is no respecter of persons. It is not an APC [All People's Congress] or SLPP [Sierra Leone People's Party] disease. It is not a disease of any political party, or ethnic group or district. Anyone who is not careful can endanger themselves and others that they love. These are extraordinary times, and extraordinary times require extraordinary measures.

This was one of several lockdowns declared in the city during the Ebola state of emergency. From the perspective of the various national and international authorities dedicated to the official Ebola response—collectively assembled under the National Ebola Response Centre—lockdowns presented an opportunity for homes to be systematically monitored for Ebola cases. The discovery of a potential case, evidenced by illness or death, generated a call to the 117 emergency service. The 117 service would coordinate with medical personnel and burial teams, all trained in Ebola safety protocol. A positive Ebola test triggered a twenty-one-day quarantine, the incubation period of the virus. Lockdowns, optimistically branded as "stay at home," were also opportunities for intensive sensitization programs, known as *os to os* (house to house), whereby residents were given basic information about identifying Ebola symptoms and the now legally enshrined protocols for informing the authorities. After households had been monitored, they were marked above the door with a series of numbers and letters in chalk. In a more general sense, lockdowns issued the message "this is an emergency."

The president's message hit home but not exactly in the ways that I had envisaged. Rather than waking up in a tense environment of people imprisoned in their homes or paralyzed by fear of the deadly outbreak that had not yet penetrated into the neighborhood, I woke up hearing my neighbors exchanging holiday greetings to each other, as they might do at Eid, Easter, or on Independence Day. As my neighbor Auntie Susan commented on seeing my reaction, "families and neighbors are all forced to spend time together around the home." This was something that in everyday life could be carefully managed. Another neighbor recounted a joke posted on a WhatsApp thread in which a young man realized that the lockdown was the new holiday when a girl asked him for her "lockdown" (i.e., a holiday gift, as might be received on Christmas or New Year's). The National Power Authority had arranged for electricity to be provided for the full three days. This was much more consistent than the norm when blackouts were daily occurrences, sometimes lasting for weeks at a time. Movement was restricted not to individual homes but rather to areas within a residential neighborhood's side streets and paths. Beyond these, the major roads were dead quiet, an inversion of the usual bustle of morning city traffic.

Taking center stage during the lockdown was an aid distribution from the local mosque, which was a major talking point among my neighbors. Hundreds of bags of rice and plastic containers of oil, donated by an international charity, were collected in the mosque's gated courtyard, which was being guarded and monitored by local city authorities and police. For much of the day there was a long line outside of members of households who had received tickets from the authorities in surveys of the neighborhood conducted ahead of the lockdown. The houses that were prioritized in this distribution were those in the newer area of the neighborhood closer to base of the valley, many of which are built from temporary materials and deemed poorer. I was struck when one young man, walking out of the mosque with a bag of rice over his shoulder, exclaimed loudly to me and a few others that "this is the first time I have benefited from APC [the ruling party] in eight years." As some disgruntled neighbors living in the older higher-up part of the neighborhood pointed out, though, it was not as if the upper part of the neighborhood was fabulously wealthy. As the afternoon progressed, the line, which seemed to be moving ever more slowly in the beating sun, grew restless until eventually, amid much shouting and discord, the gates of the mosque slammed shut.

An older woman who ran several small businesses in the city commented to me that "they [the authorities] will be back later after dark. Bend bend business [corruption] works at all levels." She was not, however, unsympathetic: "So many jobs get paid so little here, and you have to pay for transport and everything, so it is not possible to build up any other way here." Perhaps she could relate, as her break in business had come during the Sierra Leone Civil War when she informally bought and sold goods in aid shipments. "The system is working through *sababu* [connections/luck], not just through need. For some it is harder to get food than for others," explained another neighbor who did not receive a distribution. Some residents who did receive shared their portions with unlucky neighbors. I witnessed one young woman in a home that I visited regularly in the less established part of the neighborhood carefully measuring out the bag of rice and the carton of oil into four equal portions for her immediate neighbors who had not received distributions. This was a striking contrast with the usually much less quantified and more protracted mode of sharing and reciprocating between these neighbors.

The fact that food was itself so central is worthy of comment. On one level, this points to a reality in which surviving Ebola went beyond avoiding contact with the virus or receiving appropriate treatment. Survival also meant being able to eat and to share, which in many cases meant providing for dependents and proximate others. Ebola did not introduce these demands but in some cases did exacerbate them. Loss of employment, closure of produce markets, and restrictions on travel and trade were all contributing factors. On another level, food was a way of thinking about and making sense of the emergency. My neighbors' responses to the distribution were mixed. Some complained about the corruption that they saw, whereby established public authorities were abusing their influence to profit for themselves and, inevitably, their own networks of dependents. Others celebrated being public beneficiaries in ways that they were not accustomed to. This included the residents of the less established part of the neighborhood who were prioritized in the survey and the young man leaving the mosque who celebrated being a beneficiary of the government for the first time and perhaps being deemed a breadwinner when he got home.

Uniting this flurry of activity around food during the lockdown was people's collective orientation toward different dimensions of ordinary life. I suspect that this was in part a response to unusual and in some ways frightening times. For the established public authorities administering the distribution, this meant leveraging their authority in order to reproduce and, arguably, reinforce existing hierarchies during a period of change and uncertainty.[1] For the more marginal social and political actors, such as the poorer residents and youths, the lockdown offered a partial glimpse into what a more idealized version of neighborhood life could look like: a well-resourced and benevolent state that was able to provide reliable electricity and material assistance to those in need, not just those with connections, combined with more equitable and transparent relationships between neighbors. Ebola had rendered these values a national priority, as the opening line of the president's speech made clear: "Everybody in every house in every community in this country is very important."

The president was half correct in the final line of his speech: "These are extraordinary times, and extraordinary times require extraordinary measures." The times were extraordinary, but the measures in this case were not. Rather, they were in different ways remarkably ordinary. As discussed in chapter 1, a number of the core epidemiological techniques of the official Ebola response were in keeping with British colonial approaches to the Great Influenza epidemic almost a century earlier. Equally, the visibility of international aid was not new. NGOs and international organizations have been a mainstay in Freetown in the decades following the civil war in the 1990s and early 2000s. Yet, the Ebola measures did have an unusual flavor to them nonetheless. That the lockdown presented a stage for heightened scrutinizing of the practices of public authorities and family life by my neighbors was in part caused by the fact that everyone involved was primed to experience those three days as a somewhat unusual event. This chapter explores what I call the "extraordinary ordinary," referring to the unusual openings for prized notions of ordinary life to unfold during emergencies particularly for those for whom crisis of one sort or another is more the norm rather than the exception.

The Extraordinary Ordinary

"New normal" was a global buzzword during the COVID-19 pandemic as people around the world experienced lockdown for the first time. For many, the pandemic entailed more time at home than they were used to. Arrangements in workplaces, schools, and colleges changed, which allowed some to work and study at home. The abrupt halting of people's normal patterns of socialization and daily routines caused significant anxiety and distress. Those used to certain securities faced a more conditional, contingent, and precarious existence. Hospitals were overstretched, and doctors were forced to make difficult decisions about who should be given ventilators. For such people, the new normal was perhaps more accurately the new abnormal.

For others, however, the new normal was actually not that new at all. Rather, it was in many respects an old normal. A vast number of the world's population do not enjoy reliable health care. Working from home is not unfamiliar to those who perform domestic labor on a daily basis, particularly women. Epidemics and official responses to them can in many cases reenforce old normal challenges.[2] For many of Freetown's residents, Ebola was a little closer to this model. However, as we shall see, there is more to the story than the reenforcing of preexisting inequalities and challenges.

My friends and neighbors in the Congo Town neighborhood did not take Ebola lightly. Families set up chlorine handwashing stations at the entrance to their homes. Deaths in the community were typically reported to the authorities according to official protocol. But at the same time, they did not exceptionalize and prioritize Ebola in quite the same way that the global health intervention demanded. Ebola was unknown and frightening, but it was still not the most dangerous life-threatening disease at large. Routine illnesses such as malaria and typhoid continued to be deadly, perhaps even more so due to the enforced closure of many local clinics and pharmacies. Ongoing challenges in securing livelihoods, supporting dependents, and moving through the life course in a dignified way persisted.

As I have already outlined, when Freetown residents talked about Ebola, it tended to index something much more expansive than a novel disease. For example, as will be expanded on in chapter 5, when someone died and received an official Ebola burial—the protocol for all deaths during the outbreak regardless of cause—they were Ebola victims even if it was clear and medically proven that they had died from another cause. When young people complained about Ebola, they were often referring to loss of livelihood, boredom, and lack of adequate health care, features of life that were all too familiar. When someone materially benefited from Ebola aid packages or employment in the official response, they were described as eating Ebola money.[3]

On one level, the term Ebola referred to a wide array of aspects of life and death in the time of Ebola, many of them byproducts of an epidemiologically focused intervention and state of emergency. On another level, "Ebola" was a new way of talking about and responding to the short-comings and possibilities of ordinary life in Sierra Leone. This was a striking juxtaposition to media and official discourses around Ebola that emphasized what was exceptional and extraordinary about it. As I came to understand, this orientation toward ordinary life was not despite the uncertainties of the emergency or the very real dangers of the Ebola virus but rather, in some important respects, because of it.

The concepts of ordinary and normal are, of course, multifaceted. Do the terms "ordinary" and "normal" index a reality or an ideal, and if so, whose?[4] In Sierra Leone, this question was particularly pronounced during the 1991–2002 civil war. While bodily violence of war was shocking and thus televisable, it obscured the structural violence embedded in cruel and arbitrary systems of governance that have persisted as the norm from the time of colonial rule.[5] Furthermore, love—a locally specific means of positively rendering personal relationships—permeated the activities of many of those caught up in the conflict in ways that actually exceeded what was normally possible.[6] In the aftermath of war while international agencies attempted to re-create a prewar normal, more in line with statistical average, farming communities sought an "ought to be" normal rather than a return to a deeply challenging situation.[7] Following these insights from wartime in Sierra Leone, I emphasize here that ordinary life must be understood not simply as a manifestation of what life ordinarily looked like but rather as a response to being confronted with somewhat extraordinary circumstances.

On one level, responding in this kind of way might be understood as a reaction to the uncertainties and urgencies of the emergency. Doing and being preoccupied with ordinary things or attempts, especially by more privileged actors to reinforce ordinary hierarchies, were in part a way of creating a comforting sense of order. Such a response has been noted particularly in the face of war, where a focus on the maintenance of everyday social relations works to normalize life in a context of rapid change and uncertainty.[8]

But as an epidemic, Ebola in Freetown differed in some important respects from wartime even if people would sometimes connect the two. During Ebola, authority was unusually centralized within unusually well-resourced state apparatuses, as opposed to the fragmented authority often found in conflict zones. The front lines of the epidemic were not battlefields, city streets, or insurgent encampments but instead were the intimate spheres of the home and the family. It was within these domains of care that transmission typically took place but also where flexible and adaptive support was generally received in a climate of lockdowns and curfews. Crucially and perhaps in common with some conflicts, the Ebola emergency was understood as distinctly temporary, with attention placed in an unusually collective way on the near future, the unknown point at which the crisis would be declared over.

For those already facing some degree of ongoing crisis, such as youths and young adults living in precarious circumstances with few foreseeable possibilities of fulfilling their own desires to start families and progress along the life-course, the temporary yet unfolding time of emergency—with its renewed configurations of family and state—was imbued with unusual promise for enacting unrealized ideals of ordinary life, or the extraordinary ordinary. The extraordinary ordinary was a new normal that tended to reflect young people's long-term priorities. It was simultaneously ordinary in the sense of centering on the day-to-day domains of work, home, and family and was extraordinary, first by being realizable due to the unusual conditions of a global emergency and second by being prized by the actors involved and requiring careful adaptation, creativity, and negotiation between established and novel ways of doing in order to enact. As we have explored, young people in Freetown lives are largely defined by the necessity of navigating between different overlapping and social orders. In chapter 3 these were the logics of kinship and business in and around the home. In chapter 2 these were the competing expectations around workers recruited into the official Ebola response. During emergencies such as Ebola, the fact of the existence of different materially unequal social orders becomes unavoidable—expressed in the notion of two worlds discussed in chapter 1—rather than murky and buried beneath the surface. The extraordinary ordinary thus refers to the unusual clarity and possibilities that emergencies present to ordinary people. To illustrate this further, I now turn back to James, the eldest son in the Bangura family we met in chapter 3, and his girlfriend Aisha, who was pregnant for the first time during the height of the Ebola state of emergency.

Life-Crisis Ritual

It was a rainy evening two months after the three-day lockdown described at the beginning of this chapter. The state of emergency had been in effect for almost a year. By now the rate of Ebola transmission was on the way down, but weariness seemed to be growing. Every evening there was a radio announcement of the number and location of new cases and the number of deaths countrywide. I had listened to the announcement with some neighbors in the Cole compound—including Brima, the young police officer we met in chapter 3—who had gathered for an ad hoc bachelor's eve celebration; one of the group was getting married the next day, despite regulations on such gatherings. At that point several days had passed with no new cases identified locally, but the daily announcement brought the unwelcome news of a handful of new cases upcountry. The state of emergency was set to be lifted after forty-two hours had elapsed with no new cases coming to light (double the incubation period of the virus). The clock had been reset.

The party was taking place on a much smaller scale than might normally have been expected. Gatherings of more than ten people were now illegal, although many people paid off the police in order to bypass this law. But the groom was short of money. We had made a collection for a crate of locally brewed bottles of Guinness stout. One neighbor who worked for the National Power Authority had used his influence to secure electricity for our area so that we would have light and could dance to an R&B, Afrobeat, and Reggae playlist put together by James. James Bangura, usually the first to dance and crack a joke, was uncharacteristically quiet and contemplative, sitting by himself on the veranda. Brima, the police officer, explained that "James is feeling the effects of Aisha being close to giving birth."

Aisha and James, who were in their midtwenties, had been together for about two years. Aisha became pregnant shortly after the declaration of the state of emergency in 2014. The couple speculated that they conceived during one of the early lockdowns.[9] She was studying business management and finance at college, but the college had been closed until further notice during Ebola.[10] Aisha was very entrepreneurial. She set up a small shop in a makeshift room adjacent to her mother's veranda and sold everyday household items such as canned food, biscuits and sweets, mosquito-repellent coils, powdered milk, tea, and soap, which she would buy downtown in bulk. Aisha would go once a month to the *luma*, a produce market out of town, where she would buy palm oil and rice to sell, both to stock her own shop and sometimes also on behalf of her father, who had a small farm out of town. James, who worked at a restaurant and guesthouse in a nearby neighborhood, would spend much of his free time between these places of business. Aisha ran several *esusu* (rotating credit association) schemes, each with slightly different financial structures (varying sums and varying intervals of collection and distribution). Aisha's mother had a stall in the local food market, and many of her fellow market women were in Aisha's *esusu*. James had invested several hundred dollars in her shop, and equally Aisha had recently contributed to James's sister's wedding expenses, both of which bound them together as a couple looking toward a shared future. At this point, however, James was out of work. The restaurant and guesthouse that he worked at, which catered mainly to international customers, had suspended its operations because of the Ebola emergency.

Brima's comment about James's worry over Aisha's pregnancy was perceptive. As James and I arrived back at his family compound, Aisha was sitting on the veranda of the house belonging to James's uncle and aunt, Samuel and Susan. The two of them were both standing close by, alongside two of Aisha's close female friends from the neighborhood. Aisha was in severe pain. Her feet were swollen, and she could barely walk without assistance. A few hours earlier she had gone to the NGO-run maternity clinic where she had registered earlier in her pregnancy, but they told her that she was not close enough to delivering and sent her home. James suggested going to Connaught Hospital—one of Freetown's main hospitals—but this idea was rejected. Aisha had attempted to enroll in its maternity ward several weeks earlier but had not found the process easy; the state hospitals were severely overstretched during the epidemic and were also deemed hotspots for Ebola transmission, which made people hesitant to go. Instead, Aisha and her friends headed to Aisha's family compound, a few hundred meters down a steep path into the valley, where her mother was preparing for a traditional *sara* (small ceremony) that aimed to bring about an auspicious delivery. They had decided to go to a local mami, an old lady and former nurse, who would deliver the baby at her home using a combination of Western procedures and customary methods. James and his aunt Susan were particularly unhappy about this option. James told us that "they do not have much faith in that family; Christians do not make *sara*." Aisha's family was Muslim, although Aisha had started attending church with James's sisters. Susan agreed: "We wait for God to intervene." I asked if God was intervening now, and they laughed. Uncle Samuel advised James against interfering further: "This is women's business." The tension and uncertainty weighed heavily on us all, exacerbated by the fact that this was Aisha's first birth. According to Auntie Susan, "If you have more experience you can give birth at home, but if you panic you may need a caesarean, and they can't be trusted to do that."

James went to his pastor to pray privately with him, as is routine for fathers before childbirth. On Susan's instruction and against her husband's advice, we called a friend in the neighborhood, a taxi driver, who drove Susan and me to the *mami*'s house on the other side of the valley, which was experiencing a blackout at the time. The mami was frail, and it seemed as though she had been drinking that evening. Based on Aisha's swollen feet, the *mami* had deduced that she would require special treatment and was therefore prepared to refer her to the formal medical authorities. Susan fetched Aisha from inside, and we walked her back to the car, where they drove back to the clinic. Aisha was once again turned away despite being in severe pain and feeling as though she was ready to deliver. The following morning Kei—a neighbor of Aisha's who was married to James's adopted sister, Momi—took Aisha back to the clinic, where she was finally admitted. James was still unhappy to be out of the loop.

Later that same day, James and I met Aisha at the gates of the clinic carrying their newborn baby boy, who would be named Moses. The clinic was publicized as free for patients, but Aisha was forced to make an informal payment before she could be discharged, just as she had made a similar under-the-table payment to be registered. We returned to the neighborhood with the baby, stopping first at James's family compound and then on to Aisha's compound. The neighbors crowded around the baby, telling the couple *tenki* (thank you). The baby was taken to a room where Aisha and James had arranged for the baby and Aisha to stay, near to her family. Despite her earlier dismissive comment about traditional ceremonies, Auntie Susan performed a *sara* of rubbing salt and leaf around the umbilical cord so it would fall off in three days, and the baby was washed. Food was served, prepared by Aisha's mother and neighbors.

As result of having spent their formative years living near each other in a close-knit neighborhood, James Bangura and Aisha had many mutual friends and family. Aisha lived with her frail mother, whose immediate neighbors were Momi (James's sister by adoption) and her husband Kei. Kei and Momi were major figures in the homes of both James's and Aisha's families. Kei operated a small car mechanic business; most days he could be seen lying under rusty cars or directing a team of apprentices near the entrance to the Bangura family compound, where he parked the cars. As an authoritative male figure, Kei acted as an uncle to Aisha, whose father lived upcountry. Momi had inherited the role of head of the local women's secret society, established in the 1950s by the matriarch of the Bangura family who had initially settled in the area. As a result, Momi split much of her time between the compounds, where she was key figure in both. Foday, my first host, and his cousin and roommate Umaru (the comedian who we met in chapter 2), were old friends of James' and lived close to Aisha. They all attended the same church, and James and Umaru regularly ate food prepared in Kei and Aisha's house. This increased after Umaru began sleeping with Kadiatu, the niece of James's stepmother Leah, which as described was the source of some tension between and within the families.

Early in their relationship James described Aisha as his "best friend" and often sang her praises to me. He had her number saved in his phone as "my wife," and they would often, somewhat jokingly, text each other, calling each other names such as "the father of my child" and "the love of my life." On several occasions, however, Aisha expressed to me a concern that she wanted James to think more about their future. She wanted him to get better at saving money and not to waste it on drinking and "cheap popularity," by which she meant hanging out with friends who were not "serious about the future." She convinced him to join an *esusu* scheme, to which he paid 10,000 Le (roughly two dollars) a day. Aisha feared that James was spending money on other women. He in turn complained that she was overly jealous and suspicious, but Aisha told me that it was the wasted money that concerned her most.

Aisha wanted to build a household with James, but having grown up in Freetown, she knew all too well that men could not be relied on; she once explained to me how important it was not to become too dependent on men. However,

Aisha had to reconcile her desire for self-reliance with her desire to be a wife. As she once explained to me,

> when you are from a poor family, you need to find money in different places because men will let you down if you don't. But if you have money they will treat you better and will have to listen to you, as you won't be so reliant on them. When I was growing up, I didn't know how to cook, I would just go to school and come back and not help around the house, just sell market goods. It is only now, because of James, that I have learnt how to cook and keep the home.

In many respects, the pregnancy came at a bad time. Both James and Aisha experienced significant financial strains that coincided with the pregnancy and the declaration of the state of emergency. In response to travel restrictions in and out of the country as well as daily curfews on business activity during the crisis, the restaurant and guesthouse where James worked closed its operations; James lost his job and received little financial compensation. Aisha experienced her own financial crisis, as the *esusu* that she ran dramatically crashed. One client threatened legal action, after which Aisha ran away for several days, not telling her family or James where she had gone. In addition, the small grocery store that Aisha and James ran together struggled during this time in part because the *luma* were banned under state of emergency regulations.

James and Aisha remained unmarried, which made honorable family formation challenging. James attempted to "lay kola" for Aisha. This is the traditional or country method of marriage in which the husband and his family give a bride price—symbolic and monetary gifts (including kola nuts)—to the bride and her family at an engagement ceremony. The initial meeting between the families, however, was not fruitful. James complained that Aisha's family was asking too much for the bride price, not taking account of Ebola or its impact on the ways he had previously supported Aisha. Some of Aisha's friends were also critical of her family. As one female friend put it, "They should not treat her like meat for sale; that is old-fashioned thinking." Aisha's family also failed to offer to prepare food for the engagement ceremony, a traditional obligation of the bride's family. James was a "stranger" entering the household—despite in practice being a neighbor and a regular visitor—and therefore formally required hospitality. James called a meeting with his family to seek advice about whether he should attempt to renegotiate, but his father advised him strongly against making another offer, since that would bring shame on his family. Aisha told me later that she had not wanted her family to offer to prepare food for the event even on a modest scale. She feared that this would lead to even greater embarrassment down the road when they failed to mobilize the resources required to put to-gether a wedding on the grand scale considered appropriate.

By the time Aisha gave birth the couple was still unmarried, and there were no wedding plans in the pipeline. This contributed further to the instability around their son's birth and its immediate aftermath; parental roles and respon-sibilities were not clearly defined. Perhaps for this reason, Aisha and James organized a large-scale *pulnador* (baby naming ceremony, literally bring outside), which was performed two weeks after the birth. Traditionally this ritual would have been performed one week earlier, symbolizing the new arrival's first out-ing and introduction to the community. A name would be given to the baby dur-ing the ceremony, which was often administered by an elder or a religious leader. Following this tradition, James and Aisha arranged a small ceremony a week after the birth, administered by James's uncle Samuel, who was a respected schoolteacher. But they also spent an additional week arranging a much bigger public ceremony. This was challenging not just because of their financial situa-tion but also in legal terms. State of emergency bylaws prohibited gatherings of more than ten people, although at this point, approaching the end of the first year, the rules were beginning to relax. Using connections with the local police station via their neighbor Brima from the Cole compound, James and Aisha were able to secure a uniformed police presence at the ceremony, thus giving it the required semblance of legality.

Hundreds of people were invited, including significant figures such as James's former boss at the restaurant and guesthouse who made a financial contribu-tion. James was relieved that the relationship had not died; in fact, the pulnador had proved to be a vehicle for keeping it alive. Aisha invited members of the Mus-lim youth group to which she had belonged before she had converted to Chris-tianity, James's religion. Many of the guests were mutual friends and neighbors from the neighborhood. The event took place in an open space behind James's family compound under a tarpaulin. They carefully arranged rented chairs in neat rows around the small square. Fresh ginger ale was served to the guests while they waited for the ceremony to begin. The ceremony was overtly Chris-tian; proceedings were led by the pastor of a church that James had recently started attending. Hymns were sung, verses from the Bible were read, and the pastor delivered a sermon during which he commented that childhood should be taken more seriously in Sierra Leone, given that people are "once an adult, but twice a child." He spoke about how parents often start to neglect their children after a few years and commented disapprovingly on the fact that many Sierra Leoneans have children out of wedlock, as was the case for Aisha and James. The pastor added, however, that "God would judge the parents according to how they raised their child." This was a welcome and comforting message. The sermon was followed by the official naming of the baby, whom Aisha held in her arms as guests came and placed money in her lap, as is customary. Afterward, food prepared by James's sisters and stepmother Leah was served on disposable plates. It was the type of food, often called "white food," that is typically served at wedding receptions: jollof rice, noodles, prawn crackers, and balls of beef. All of these features of the ceremony—the food, the religious aspects, and the scale—were more reminiscent of a Christian wedding ceremony than a typical pulnador.

The fact that the baby naming ceremony resembled a modern wedding was not coincidental; it seemed to be a self-conscious substitute created by Aisha and James as an attempt to present a positive public image as they set about starting their own family. The life-course ritual itself involved improvisation and adaptation alongside conservative, traditional features. The pulnador was delayed for a week and took place on a much larger scale than would normally have been the case. At the same time, the embrace of a respected family ritual, in which a baby is honorably accepted into a community, was a significant nod toward tradition. The ceremony thus represented an alignment and fulfillment of intergenerational expectations pertaining to social reproduction. Conversely, the ceremony reflected the tension between generational hierarchies and in this respect had an almost antiauthoritarian bent to it. After all, Aisha's parents had not agreed to James's initial request for marriage, deeming the payment too small. And James's family had advised him against renegotiation, with its risk of further humiliation. It was notable that Aisha's parents were not present at the ceremony and nor was James's father, who remained in his room. His absence was attributed to his frailty at the time, and he was indeed ill. The ceremony occurred while James and Aisha lacked formal employment, so money and other resources were in short supply. But the ceremony helped to establish a network of support around the baby, all the more valuable given the uncertain circumstances into which he had been born. And James's inclusion of his former boss from the job he had lost during the Ebola emergency helped to reestablish an important relationship with a patron that the epidemic had jeopardized.

Ebola clearly presented serious obstacles to the social acknowledgment of movement through the life course. But for young people, challenges surrounding the life course were not novel.[11] In Sierra Leone, with one of the highest rates of child and maternal mortality globally, pregnancy and birth are always risky regardless of whether there is a global health emergency. On top of this, as has been well documented in scholarship in recent decades and discussed in previous chapters, African youths face widespread difficulties in participating as central actors in life-course rituals and family-based social reproduction and, in related ways, achieving social adulthood. Although many young people in Freetown have children, they struggle to start their own families in honorable and widely accepted ways. As James and Aisha's case exemplified, this was often not because of being disconnected from family, as is often suggested in crisis of youth scholarship, but instead because of being greatly and complexly interconnected, making it challenging to untangle and realign intimacies necessary for honorable family formation. Additionally, it was difficult for many of those whose family straddled town and country to find the right balance between meeting both modern urban and traditional rural expectations.

Therefore, Ebola landed in a place in which social reproduction was already in crisis. For those stuck or marginal in family networks, the emergency—including regulations explicitly targeting family rituals—did not necessarily impede rituals' efficacy. In fact, traditional ritual seemed to be injected with heightened potency and possibility for young people. It is perhaps fitting that an emergency would be productive of ritual. Ritual-based social reproduction—even at its most ideal—is a crisis-ridden process, hence the term "life crisis" used by some anthropologists as a synonym for life course or life cycle with reference to ritual. Ritual, as an event, typically comes as a break in the normal flow of social life and is often infused with an atmosphere of urgency and regulation, which participants relate to in heightened and personal ways, what Victor Turner calls "the subjunctive mood."[12] In the rhythm of family life in Freetown, the greatest demands are often made in the buildup to and during rituals. It is at these times—especially around sickness and death and birth and marriage—that the need for material support, or for people to show up, is most potent. During Ebola when officially sanctioned adaptation to rituals was under way, ritual gained renewed meaning for youths in part due to the greater possibility they found for their own adaptations.

The baby naming ceremony was illegal under state of emergency regulations, given restrictions on gatherings of over ten people. But for the participants it remained a priority, which cannot be written off as frivolous or uniformed. Rather, the ceremony reflects a reality in which social life continued despite and in some senses because of Ebola, a case of the extraordinary ordinary. Surviving Ebola was not only a matter of avoiding contagion or receiving treatment but was also a broader social matter of getting through the emergency in an honorable and meaningful way. The family and the home were the primary targets of official security-focused regulation and scrutiny, which resulted in people often being forced to spend more time at home and with family than they were used to. Family-based rituals were thus an appropriate form for young people to enact meaningful transformation during the emergency. The urgent and temporary albeit unfolding and uncertain qualities of the emergency were harnessed by young people in pursuing their own projects of honorable family formation. Although regulations presented obstacles, these could be creatively overcome, as James and Aisha found out. However, the fact that during the emergency family rituals, particularly burials, were being intentionally regulated and reshaped by authorities, in line with epidemiological priorities as well as some adherence to tradition, made it more acceptable and possible for ordinary people do so too, in line with their own priorities.

For James and Aisha these priorities were at once short-term, in securing a safety net around their newborn son, and long-term, in gaining public recognition of their new family. By adapting a traditional baby naming ceremony to serve as a modern wedding, they were able to attend to these priorities. In doing so, they were enacting established practices in Freetown of navigating between different social orders, following on from the Krio, the decedents of the former British and American slaves who founded the city in the late eighteenth century and brokered between local and British colonial orders during the colonial period, outlined in chapter 1. In Freetown, the Krio present an enduring model for those of different ethnic backgrounds—such as for James's and Aisha's families who were from indigenous Sierra Leonean groups—of how ritual and ceremony are used to maintain familial networks, which are central for surviving different scales of crisis and emergency. But James and Aisha were also drawing on their more immediate personal experience of navigating the social expectations of kinship and business, described in chapter 3, in the intimate spaces of the home and family. The Ebola emergency presented openings whereby coexisting yet contradictory social orders were more clearly delineated by those caught up in them, which allowed for them to be creatively realigned.

In a well-known essay, Jane Guyer describes a global temporal shift in the early twenty-first century—reflected in both neoliberal economic and Pentecostal religious thinking—in which the near future is "evacuated."[13] Without medium-term predictability and continuity, collective attention is instead focused on the immediate present and a long-term, somewhat fantastical, future. This would relatively accurately describe much of the life that I and other researchers observed among young people in Sierra Leone pre-Ebola. In the time of Ebola, however, young people's relationship to the near future was transformed in some important respects. Although the near future remained uncertain, it did occupy a great deal of collective attention.[14] In chapter 2 we saw how for those employed in the official Ebola response, the near future was a space that was reinhabited in interconnected ways by formal employment, personal life projects, new solidarities, and the keeping up of family commitments.[15] The near future was a national preoccupation as the rate of new Ebola cases was continually monitored, which ultimately determined how long the state of emergency would be in place. In other words, there was an unusual sense of continuity between activities in the present and the imagined future.

It was within this temporary yet unfolding time of emergency that the extraordinary ordinary—the unusual openings for prized notions of ordinary life during crises—could play out. But this was not a given; it required careful attentiveness and negotiation, as pitfalls were plentiful. This chapter explored the extraordinary ordinary during several events: a neighborhood lockdown, a birth, and a baby naming ceremony. Each of these events were in different ways conditioned by the state of emergency and international humanitarian intervention, featuring novel regulations on family life and material flows. But these events reveal young people's agency in shaping the emergency in line with their own priorities and ideals. Although ongoing challenges and inequalities did not disappear and were in some cases exacerbated by the official Ebola response, young people discovered transformative potential in a number of the features of the emergency, including: the transformed state and family, the atmosphere of urgency, collective attention on the near future, the unusual capacity for family ritual to be adapted, and the unusual clarity on the existence of multiple social orders in day-to-day life.

These transformations were significant because of the ways they contrasted and interacted with the deep-rooted, slow-burning crisis that young people in Freetown as well as across the continent and the globe face in realizing inherited and personal ideals and expectations, in particular notions of personhood and maturity based on the ability to start families, find jobs, and receive recognition and support from elders and the state. In chapter 5, we look at another crisis that befell the Bangura family, although this time at other end of the life course.

BLACK AND WHITE DEATH

On the afternoon of August 6, 2015, I received a text message from James Bangura: "Auntie Marie's condition is bad, and she has been admitted to the hospital and is in the isolation ward."

As described in chapter 4, James Bangura and Aisha held a naming ceremony for their newborn son during Ebola. Despite state of emergency regulations on gatherings and difficulties in securing funds during the emergency, the young couple found unusual meaning and possibility in a traditional yet adapted life-course ritual. This chapter examines ritual at the other of the life course. Only a few months before the baby naming ceremony, James's family—who were hosting me in their family compound at the time—were in the midst of another life crisis.[1] Marie, the sister of James's stepmother Leah (whom we first met in chapter 3), had come to live in the compound after her speedy marriage to a visiting diasporic Sierra Leonean and German national. Months after his return to Europe, Marie unexpectedly died due to pregnancy complications. How were the family to honor and grieve Marie when a traditional burial and funeral were now strictly prohibited due to risks of Ebola transmission?

Funerals during the Ebola epidemic were unusually heightened occasions. Those close to the deceased faced expected emotional and logistical challenges after loss that were often intensified when confronted with the demands of the public health intervention. Regulation of burials was one of the five key pillars of the official Ebola response. This made burials almost emblematic of the emergency as a whole. At the same time, activity around death often has a heightened feel to it. In Freetown while proximity to death in close-knit and poorly serviced communities is almost a predictable part of day-to-day life, the performance of appropriate funerary practices remains perhaps the most revered of social obligations.

Such attitudes to burial can be ascribed to not only belief systems that emphasize the dynamic relationship between the world of the living and the dead but also the day-to-day practices of family life and maintenance. Abner Cohen, who did fieldwork with Freetown Krio families in the 1960s and 1970s, expressed it like this: "To put it bluntly, your 'family' consists of the persons who come, with presents and contributions in hand, to eat, drink, or grieve in your ceremonials."[2] Anthropologists have long attended to the ways that "good death" is enacted socially through the performance of appropriate funerary ritual. Good death is not only an act of care for the deceased but is also often understood as a key process through which social order among the living is restored in the aftermath of loss.[3] Conversely, "bad death" can create crisis in its own right.[4]

During the Ebola epidemic, securing good death by traditional standards was particularly challenging. Since the corpses of Ebola victims are highly contagious, there is considerable risk of transmission during funerals through ritual body washing and contact between mourners. During the early stages of the outbreak, bodies were left in the street, and mortuaries overflowed. Not surprisingly, then, burial practices became highly regulated by national and international authorities within the state of emergency. Regardless of the Ebola status of the deceased—and the majority of deaths during the emergency were not caused by the disease—all burials were legally supposed to be performed by official burial teams, often in purpose-built cemeteries.

Burial teams—such as Peter's team described in chapter 2—were staffed primarily by young men working under the auspices of the Ministry of Health and international NGOs. The teams were trained and equipped to perform all burials according to an unfamiliar biomedical paradigm featuring clinical management and strict procedures oriented toward safety and efficiency. But efforts were made to incorporate elements of traditional burial practice, such as allowing up to ten mourners and religious leaders to be present. Both priorities were encapsulated in the slogan "safe and dignified burials." For home deaths, family members were required to call the 117 emergency service, which would coordinate with a burial team stationed in the vicinity to collect the body within twenty-four hours. If the death occurred in a medical facility, staff would coordinate with the team. Freetown was divided into four bases, with about twenty teams serving the city. The teams were initially managed by the Ministry of Health, but in October 2014 many of the responsibilities of managing, recruiting, training, and funding were handed over to NGOs. By early 2015 after more funding, training, and new management, the burial teams became proficient at performing their duties like clockwork, as an international manager once told me.

Some people tried to avoid these regulations altogether, choosing to perform illegal secret burials, in which, for example, they would bury in chosen neighborhood cemeteries and family plots rather than at new unfamiliar Ebola cemeteries. Secret burials, while technically illegal under state of emergency bylaws, were often arranged in coordination with established public authorities such as the police, the city council, and the military (as opposed to the novel burial teams) also though at the risk of a hefty punishment.

Burials therefore presented an apparent tension between established ways of dealing with death and efficient epidemic management. Below the surface was a conflict between, on one hand, the expectations of authorities and recruits within the international public health intervention and state of emergency and, on the other hand, those of established public authorities and communities on the ground. In rural settings in particular, this conflict was often insurmountable. Official burial teams sometimes encountered active resistance from village communities[5] or, in less overt ways, intruded in and undermined the effectiveness of local efforts at safe burial.[6] In Freetown, however, conflict around management of the dead was met with considerable amounts of negotiation and compromise. This chapter in part aims to explain how and why city dwellers caught up in the middle of this conflict understood its severity and yet were equipped to respond in such seemingly balanced ways.

The language that was used to describe different types of burials and death during the epidemic tells us a lot. The terminology in Freetown was strikingly racial. Broadly speaking, the official Ebola burials that were performed by the burial teams were unofficially dubbed "white" death. Secret burials, by contrast, were known as "black" death, being more aligned to customary practices. Yet, the differences were not, as might be expected, black and white. Rather, the boundaries between black and white death were porous and often blurry. Secret burials were more private than many normal Freetown burials and required extensive bureaucratic navigation and incorporation of new safety protocols. Official white burials were performed not by White foreigners but instead primarily young Black Sierra Leonean men who served as formally employed gatekeepers of the public health intervention.

"Black" and "white" are quotidian reference points in Freetown, representing primary yet complex overlapping social categories through which norms, values, and practices are understood. During the emergency these categories were destabilized and fraught—expressed in the notion of two worlds that often accompanies global health and humanitarian initiatives—and yet took on heightened explanatory value for ordinary people. The coding of burials in racial terms points to Sierra Leone's long history of integration into the Atlantic world, outlined in chapter 1. Sierra Leone was the primary site of capture for slaves sent to

North America. Foreign intervention in Africa, going back to the slave trade and British colonialism, has always come with violent and oppressive processes of racialization, which the international intervention during Ebola could not shake off. Yet, Freetown residents were also drawing on the city's deep-rooted cosmopolitism, including its origin as a refuge for freed slaves, in which nonessentialized, flexible notions of race have rich historical precedence. They were thus able to assemble a genuinely meaningful framework for negotiating loss in the midst of an intervention and emergency.

Two Burials

Marie was a charismatic and worldly woman in her late thirties. She was the sister of James's stepmother Leah and had come to live with us a few months earlier after her marriage to a German citizen of Sierra Leonean origin, with whom she had become pregnant. Marie was preparing to join her husband, referred to in the Bangura family as "the German," in Europe, a task complicated by the Ebola emergency because Freetown's German consulate had stopped issuing visas. For Marie, the obstacles she faced reflected not only the stretching of bureaucratic channels by the regional and global crisis of Ebola but also perceived jealousies among her extended family and neighbors in Freetown. As she put it to me once, "You know, Black people, we have Black mind." It was because of these perceived jealousies that she had moved from the house where she had been living to stay with us in the Bangura family compound, where Leah lived. Marie had been unwell for several weeks. While her illness did not seem serious, it was persistent. Helped by Leah, Marie sought medical attention, but the efforts were fruitless. Finally, Marie collapsed and was taken to the Cottage Hospital in Freetown's old Fourah Bay area. The city's medical system was overstretched by Ebola; many patients were either refused admission or resisted going for fear of being (mis)diagnosed as positive for Ebola. A few hours after James sent his text message, he called to tell me that Marie had died in the hospital.

I went straight to the hospital, feeling that it was expected of me. I had often observed the importance of friends and family coming close in times of crisis. I met James, his uncle Samuel, one of his cousins, his stepbrother Kei, and a neighbor who worked as a technician in the hospital. The group was attempting to make arrangements for Marie's burial. Their efforts centered on gaining access to the body so they could perform the burial themselves; this was illegal under the state of emergency bylaws. Regardless of the deceased's Ebola status, all burials during the state of emergency were to be performed by official teams at the new NGO-managed Waterloo Cemetery in eastern Freetown. Consultations

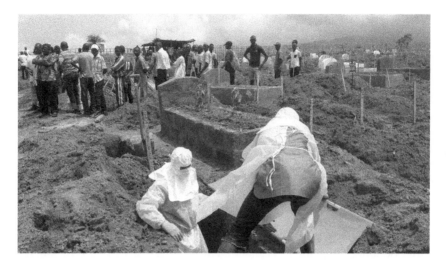

FIGURE 4.   Ebola burial team members and mourners at the Waterloo Cemetery.

with the mortuary staff made it clear that illegal access to the body in order to perform a secret burial—still common for families with the right connections and the ability to make sufficient payments—was out of the question. The body was still in the isolation ward and therefore difficult to access, especially after a recent dispute between the medical and mortuary staff over the distribution of payments.

We returned to the hospital the next morning. The test results were negative for both Ebola and malaria. There were further negotiations with hospital staff over whether Marie's body could be dressed and perfumed before the burial team took her. A family friend and former nurse at the hospital had volunteered to perform this duty dressed in personal protective equipment. The request was refused on the grounds that the "White doctors would not allow it." Instead, the body was put into a standardized body bag, carried to the white van used by the burial team to transport corpses, and taken to the Waterloo Cemetery on the outskirts of town (figure 4).

We arrived at the cemetery before the team, which had to collect other bodies on the way. Hundreds of mourners were waiting to witness burials. When our team came, we were called into the cemetery by a young man wearing tinted-blue sunglasses and a tight matching vest and shorts made of Africana fabric. He looked as though he had stepped out of a Nigerian afrobeat music video but was in fact responsible for the challenging task of coordinating the mourners, the burial teams, and cemetery staff. The young men in the team, some of whom I recognized from my research, lowered the body into the pre-dug plot assigned to

Marie. Francis, Marie's elder brother, had bought a wooden mesh that was placed over the body bag (there had been no time to make a coffin) so that dirt was not cast disrespectfully directly onto the naked body. After a short negotiation with the burial team supervisor, the body bag was opened so that the family could take one last look at Marie's face. Marie's twin brother, a filmmaker by trade, was recording the proceedings closely, partly for Marie's husband in Germany. The eight or so mourners huddled together, taking photos on their smartphones. With no pastor available and uncertain how to proceed in this unfamiliar and unusually institutionalized environment, James spontaneously took the lead. He recited the Lord's Prayer, stoically declaring, in the manner of a cleric at the graveside, that "God marks our time to die for a purpose that we don't know or understand." A metal sign was erected with Marie's personal details, including the plot number, to make it easier for the family to locate the grave in the future.

When we got back to the compound, Leah served us large plates of groundnut soup with fish and rice, which she had prepared for those who would come to *tel osh* (share their sympathies). The people who had been at the cemetery reported what they had witnessed. They spoke of the horror and cruelty of Ebola: long rows of freshly dug graves, the arrival of the burial team with thirteen bodies (a figure regularly quoted in the compound in the coming weeks), all children apart from Marie, and, perhaps most powerfully, the grave of a young woman that was being filled in with no mourners present. James admitted that this was what finally brought him to tears. At the same time, their reports sounded notes of admiration. The orderly running of the cemetery, involving independent coordination between gravediggers and the burial team (without family involvement), and the measured neatness in the arrangement of plots were by turn unfamiliar and impressive. Francis, Marie and Leah's older brother, presented Leah with a bag containing the white shawl and perfume he had bought in the hope of being able to dress Marie. This served as the necessary evidence that he had tried his hardest to bury their sister according to established norms.

Leah reflected later that "Ebola means that you don't feel it when somebody dies. They do it [the burial] so quickly, but then you will sit down and remember them, imagine about them." This profound comment seemed to crystallize the cruelty of Ebola when the pressing and emotionally charged obligations surrounding death became entangled with the imposing presence of a novel public health intervention. The immediacy of the Ebola emergency and present-oriented pressures to fight it were difficult to square with the enduring feeling of obligations surrounding good death in Sierra Leone, in which the deceased's eternal fate lay in the balance.

Soon after hearing that Marie had died, James's cousin asked fearfully whether she might have had Ebola and was sharply criticized by other family members for expressing self-concern at an inappropriate time. It was not that the risk of catching Ebola was not taken seriously—many of those in the compound were taking precautions against it and were critical of those who did not—but that fear of infection, at least on paper, was considered temporary and individual compared to the obligations that arose from the death of a close family member or friend. As Peter, the motorbike taxi rider and burial team worker, once put it to me, "In Sierra Leone we care about the person more once they have died than when they are alive."

There was a powerful atmosphere of unresolved anxiety in the compound in the weeks after Marie's death reflecting the incompleteness of her life—her pregnancy and planned migration to Europe—and the uncertainty about the cause of her death. This was compounded by the incompleteness of the funerary rites. Burial teams were tasked with performing burials on the same day that the body was collected, which created significant time pressures for mourners. Muslim burials in Freetown are typically performed soon after the death; following the ritual washing and wrapping of the body in a *lapa* (sheet), there is a procession from the local mosque or house of the deceased to the cemetery. Christian burials often take place weeks after a death, leaving time to prepare a coffin, *kasanka* (special clothes for the corpse), badges with pictures of the deceased, personalized service booklets, and food and drink. A *wekin* (vigil) is usually held the night before the burial, followed by a church service in the morning and a procession to the cemetery, often involving uniformed bands. At times, bodies are transported from Freetown to natal villages for burial in family plots alongside prominent ancestors. Restrictions on gatherings made Muslim memorial services—typically on the first, third, fourth, and fortieth days after the death—challenging to perform. The handling of corpses was prohibited for risk of infection, and this precluded the ritual washing of bodies, performed at home or in mortuaries, as well as the ceremonies conducted by secret societies after their members pass away.

In Sierra Leone, the treatment of the dead—including those responsible for performing key tasks and the manner and locations in which burials are performed—are closely connected to the status of the deceased. Burials are key means through which claims to land are made, especially in rural contexts, and it is through respectable burial in the presence of elders that the link between the ancestors and the living is maintained and that blessings for the community secured. Funerals and memorial services are also important opportunities for family meetings, at which disputes are voiced and settled in the presence of elders and stakeholders. Negotiations often included the care of dependents of the deceased and distribution of the deceased's property.[7] Burial teams, however, were trained to be blind to the status of the deceased and their families, ensuring the use of the same type of body bags, the same cemetery, and the same treatment for all. Thus, Ebola was seen as presenting a greater challenge in some cases than in others.

This did not, however, preclude adaptation, often improvised on the ground. Marie's mourners' attempted to negotiate certain allowances at the Waterloo cemetery and afterward in the arrangements for memorialization. Immediately after her burial, Marie's family started planning a memorial service—adapted from the Muslim forty days ceremony—that would be less hampered by regulation than the burial, allowing the family to mark Marie's death in a more fitting manner. For several weeks after the death, her German husband had been uncommunicative and did not readily contribute to expenses that the family was incurring. During this period rumors, albeit hotly debated and contested, circulated in the neighborhood and beyond that the German had visited Freetown every few years, each time becoming attached to women who died soon after. In these narratives he was symbolically transformed from a well-meaning "white" European citizen who could help the family to a "black" ritualist (someone who uses witchcraft to sacrifice others for personal profit).[8]

Ultimately, Marie's burial was performed not according to traditional standards but instead according to the protocols of an all-encompassing bureaucratic system, which dictated that every person who died, regardless of whether they were among the close to the recorded four thousand Sierra Leoneans who died from Ebola, was buried as if they had contracted the disease. Although Marie tested negative, she was nevertheless buried as if she had Ebola and thus became a victim so to speak of mass death. Instead of a family plot or a local cemetery, where her body would have been interred alongside family or community members of previous generations, Marie was buried among people who had in common only that they had died during the time of Ebola. The number assigned by the burial team indicated statistically and spatially, in the neat rows of the recently established Waterloo cemetery, where Marie fell in this mass death. The community in which she was buried did not mirror the one in which she had lived but rather the time and circumstances of her death.

Since Marie died in hospital, her family had no choice but to work with the Ebola authorities. In many other cases families simply failed to report a death to the burial teams, preferring to perform burials themselves. Although referred to as secret burials, prohibited under the state of emergency and punishable by heavy fines and arrest, these funerals were not inevitably deemed illegal; they resulted from negotiations with established bureaucratic and legal structures that were often perceived to carry more weight than new Ebola authorities. The secret burials too were highly structured, with built-in—though far from watertight—safety measures. By means of permission, assistance, and documentation from authorities such as the Freetown City Council (who issued Ebola-free death certificates), the police and their postmortem teams (who often administered their own Ebola tests), mortuary workers, ambulance drivers, and the military, it was possible for mourners to perform burials themselves at places and times of their own choosing. Negotiating with these gatekeepers typically required large payments (roughly US$400) or high-level connections, so they were undertaken primarily, though not exclusively, when people of high status died. In my neighborhood, local representatives of the city council became experts in managing secret burials; they were already responsible for managing the local cemetery. Their most prominent project, conceived before but executed during and after the emergency, was erecting a wall around the cemetery, in part to prevent street youths from congregating there. Their authority and their connections to the city's existing bureaucratic institutions, the local community, and the cemetery meant that council members were well positioned to broker secret burials.

While the burial teams were criticized for performing burials too hastily, the secret alternatives could be too slow. In June 2015 I attended the burial of Rachel, a nurse and a prominent member of a local Pentecostal church a few minutes' walk from where I lived, who had reportedly tested negative for Ebola. Her body was being kept in the mortuary of a military hospital not too far away. Her husband, a teacher in a local school, had planned to perform the burial the previous day, when a large number of mourners had gathered at the hospital for a service, but he was unable to secure all the necessary documentation in time. The next day after permission was received and arrangements were made with council representatives for the grave to be dug in the local cemetery, Rachel's body was transported, effectively in disguise, from the mortuary to the cemetery gates in an ambulance, with military personnel accompanying as an extra security measure. The Christian practice of a *wekin* (vigil) the night before the burial at the house of the deceased was abandoned, and—inverting the usual practice—a church service was performed after the burial without the body present. Some local young men volunteered to carry the coffin to the grave after purposefully donning the disposable blue medical gloves that were handed out as an Ebola-inspired safety precaution. The ambulance hurriedly left the scene. As the body was lowered into the ground, uniformed girls from Rachel's husband's school sang a hymn. Before they had finished, the volunteers had already begun helping the regular cemetery gravediggers to fill in the grave, hoping to speed up the job. As the crowd—mostly dressed in black and white—was dispersing, a local fixer collected money to tip the gravediggers and the cemetery staff. The remaining mourners stood by, carefully observing the filling in of the grave and the collecting and counting of the money. In the heat of the midday sun, it occurred to me that the gravediggers, volunteers, and witnesses were performing two stressful tasks: burying a loved one and burying the evidence. The burial was improvised and hybrid, informed by enduring obligations of custom-ary funerary obligations yet adapted with respectful reference to the biomedi-cal norms introduced by burial teams as well as genuine acknowledgment of the risks of infection and punishment for illegal burial.

"Black" and "White" Social Orders

Marie's and Rachel's families and mourners encountered unusual obstacles along the established pathways for transforming unexpected and premature loss into good death. In the case of Marie, only a handful of mourners attended the burial, contributing to a feeling of incompleteness in the grieving process, articulated with such clarity by Leah, Marie's sister. Rachel's burial entailed unusual degrees of adaptation and caution in circumventing state of emergency bylaws. Difficul-ties in achieving good death are commonplace in emergencies, particularly in wartime.[9] But during Ebola, the centralized regulation and management of mor-tuary practices were not collateral challenges but instead were the principle aims of the internationally led public health intervention. Around death, mourn-ers came into direct contact with a defining social conflict of the emergency: "local" beliefs and practices versus those of the international response.

Yet, in Freetown and almost certainly beyond, this conflict was far from clear-cut. The simultaneous expressions of praise and horror that I heard from my fellow mourners at the Waterloo cemetery point to such ambiguity. They sug-gested that Marie's Ebola burial did not render it meaningless, even if a good death, as customarily measured, was not achieved. Equally, while Rachel's burial was technically illegal under state of emergency bylaws, it nonetheless took on new safety features and a claim to legality by virtue of having navigated an al-ternative yet arguably more established bureaucratic process involving a num-ber of public authorities. While burials during Ebola were occasions of heightened tension, conflict, and pain, they contained within them a great deal of compro-mise and flexibility.[10]

How can we account for these apparently contradictory dynamics? How did Freetown residents account for them? The coding of burials in a racial language of black and white is a major clue. These categories are used in Freetown to refer to different social orders and sets of cultural norms and values that coexist in the city and were thus a ready-made framework for making sense of death and burial during Ebola. "Black" and "white" are Sierra Leonean and in particular Freetown-centric terms for describing the types of contradictory yet porous so-cial orders that we have encountered in previous chapters: for example, the two worlds of international intervention in chapter 1, the competing expectations around involvement in the official Ebola response in chapter 2, the relational order of kinship versus the transactional order of business in the chapter 3, and tradition versus adaptation in coming-of-age ceremonies in chapter 4.

"Black," also sometimes called "African," typically refers to local culture, while "white" refers to foreign Western culture. In the white system, as it is sometimes described, people are seen to act according to fixed principles and cannot be convinced to alter their professional responsibilities. The burial teams were formally trained to adhere to this ideal, which included treating all dead bodies and mourning families the same regardless of age, status, or personal connections. In the black system, by contrast, people are viewed as showing bias toward some over others, particularly their own people (family, friends, community) and sometimes those more senior or willing to compensate appropriately.

The white and black categories are for most people both positive and negative in their valence, often depending on the circumstances. The white system might be admired as principled, fair, and necessary for development, while the black system is derided as backward, selfish, and, in a Fanon-esque way, self-destructive.[11] Yet, at other times the alternative evaluations are made, with the black system indexing enduring values such as tradition, care, and respectability as well as adaptability and resilience, while the white system is viewed as having only material and temporary value, and as oppressive and cruel. During Ebola, these opposing moral evaluations became starker than usual. The black system was represented in a dominant discourse in the official Ebola response as an obstacle to containing the outbreak. As a Sierra Leonean burial team supervisor once told me, "Black culture is the problem here." Yet, for many the positives were just as strongly felt particularly in terms of traditional commitments to care and support, which were crucial during the hard times of the emergency.

The categories of black and white are also used in Freetown to index contrasting temporal orientations, a recurring reference point throughout my fieldwork there. "White time" referenced an abstract ideal of events occurring in a predetermined and predictable manner that was often at odds with the reality of life (and death) in Freetown, which necessitates operating in "black time." Through the white lens this might be seen as being late, but through the black lens it signaled adherence to an implicit sense of the "right" time, which factored in the juggling of social obligations as well as the endless practical obstacles—broken-down cars, unavailable funds, sudden illness or death—that Freetown residents routinely navigate. Burials are a heightened case of this, where the temporal consequences include the eternal fate of the deceased and the most enduring of social and ritual obligations, yet volatile circumstances require flexibility and adaptability in the moment. As death in the time of Ebola made plain, the clockwork of white time—while exemplifying a Weberian ideal of bureaucratic order—presented a form of cruel impersonal disorder, a metronomic punctuality opposed to the comforting rhythm of activity typically associated with good death.

Alongside the discursive mobilization of the categories of black and white by my interlocutors, the categories also took on embodied forms. Anthropologists of Sierra Leone have pointed to the body as a primary site where the country's traumatic history of slavery holds enduring meaning in day-to-day movements through historically embedded landscapes and in ritual.[12] The body is also widely regarded by anthropologists as a primary locus of racialization.[13] Yet, bodily performance and embodied memory escape the limits of discourse. Not only are they particularly prone to holding violent and traumatic histories, but they also allow for flexibility and ambiguity beyond what is discursively possible. The centrality of the body in funerary ritual of both the dead and the living may explain why burials were key sites for the resurfacing of the black and the white during the emergency.[14]

In black death, the body was recognized as a member of a family and a community and would both gain safe passage to the world by coming through religiously informed ritual and receive a final claim to status among the living. Secret burials aimed to achieve this by adhering as much as possible to existing norms and to work through established, though marginalized, bureaucratic and authoritative channels. In white death the body was hazardous material, requiring specialist training to handle and dispose of safely in order to protect the corporeal world from the further spread of Ebola. Burials performed by the burial teams constituted the dead as part of a cruel mass death, in large measure because of the teams' strict adherence to uniform, biomedically informed procedures that treated all the dead as Ebola victims regardless of their cause of death.

While the black and white categories reference cultural norms and practices as well as individual and collective identities, the boundaries between each are in practice blurred and shifting in part because of their embodied as well as discursive character. As we have seen throughout this book, including in this chapter, people regularly transformed and mediated between them, seemingly taking on features of both. The gatekeeper of the Waterloo cemetery and, by extension, the white system of the official Ebola response, dressed not in the uniform of a recognizable official but instead in the black style of a *raray boy* (street youth). The permanent hospital staff would not allow access to Marie's body because of the White doctors, thus aligning themselves with institutional professionalism over influence through personal connections. The local representatives of the city council brokered secret burials, similar to pre-Ebola burials but adapted for the emergency. The German, the gatekeeper of the connection to Europe of Marie and her family, was transformed from a "white" European to a "black" representative of Freetown's illicit underworld. And perhaps my own journey as an anthropologist who was socialized by my hosts from "white" to "black," although not in any linear or stable way. In other words, the balancing of the white and black systems is required to varying degrees of all Freetown residents on a daily basis. During the emergency and the large-scale humanitarian and public health intervention that came with it, however, the black and white social orders were more in evidence and more volatile than usual.[15]

In Sierra Leone these racial categories recall a long history of violent integration into the Atlantic world, outlined in greater detail in chapter 1. Beginning in the early sixteenth century, Sierra Leone became a major site of extraction for slaves who were mostly sent to North America. Freetown was established in 1792 by immigrant free persons of color and Black Londoners after the British ban on the international slave trade, what is sometimes considered the first humanitarian project. The descendants of these founders, who were joined by waves of recaptives (Black Africans illegally held on slave ships and rescued by the Royal Navy) and migrating Black British colonial subjects, became known as the Krio, also the name of Sierra Leone's dominant spoken language, an English Creole. The Krio as an ethnic group came to be seen as simultaneously and alternately "black," through their historic link to slavery, diaspora, and colonial racism, and "white," through their sometimes elite status in Freetown, secured through identification with British imperial institutions and culture: Christian practice, small family sizes, English-sounding names, European dress, property ownership, and architectural styles that retain a distinctive presence in Freetown. The Krio thus positioned themselves as "interpreters of Western culture to other Africans,"[16] through which their elite status in the colonial administration was at times secured, although such positions equally led to racist resentment by White authorities who labeled them "savvy niggers" and "trousered Africans." While the Krio are now a minority in Freetown, their history is key to the formation of nonessentialized understandings of race in the city—within a general context of often severe racism—and in providing an enduring model of brokerage, mediation, and transformation between "black" and "white," which became starkly evident during the Ebola emergency among actors from a wide range of backgrounds.

Freetown has continued to serve as an unstable global hub in the postcolonial period, where the balancing of black and white systems is of continued significance. The civil war saw the rise of NGOs, humanitarian interventions, and internationally led liberal peace-building initiatives, along with the proliferation of human rights and development discourses. Yet, rather than eliminating distinctions between those of the black and white systems, as universalist discourses might be expected to do, these categories have in some senses been pitted against each other.[17] Critical analyses of the Ebola emergency have similarly highlighted the conflict between local culture and foreign norms or have shown how local culture was largely neglected by the international response, thus reinforcing rather than blurring the fault line between the two and forcing the marginalized to come up with creative solutions.[18]

But black and white death adds another layer to this story in which disruption to and the continuity of meaningful social processes were not mutually exclusive. On the one hand, these categories reveal violence structurally embedded within systems of global health and humanitarianism. Humanitarians might consider themselves as being blind to race by their alignment to (notably Western) notions of universal needs. But humanitarianism is in practice, of course, historically and culturally contingent. As an overtly foreign intervention, the official Ebola response was meaningful in relation to a specific regional history of coercive intervention that has been accompanied by imported notions of race. Yet, on the other hand, racial categories have become thoroughly incorporated and reworked into meaningful conceptual frameworks and ways of getting by and through the life course in Freetown. In this process, they have taken on a degree of fluidity that differs from the more fixed, essentialized understandings of race that are commonplace in the West. While they do connote what is distinct—and opposed—between different social orders, they also contain within them the possibility for creative brokerage.

Marie's and Rachel's unexpected deaths, like that of many others during the epidemic, tore at the fabric of the family and the community. Mourners' attempts to deal with their losses were complicated by a public health intervention in which regulation and management of death and burial was a priority. Challenges in enacting good death—a principle means of maintaining and reproducing social order in the face of disorder—redefined not only responses to death during Ebola but also experiences of the emergency more broadly. Official Ebola burials were a key component of the epidemiological response, yet it was those same burial practices that constituted those who received them—a far greater number than those who died from the disease—as part of the mass death of Ebola in mourner's eyes. Understandably, if you were buried like an Ebola victim, then you were an Ebola victim.

Freetown residents, however, were not working with a singular notion of order in their approaches to good death and burial but instead were drawing on two social "orders": black and white. It was not simply that white order represented disorder, although the conflict was acknowledged in this language. Rather, both simultaneously represented order and disorder for residents. Buried beneath these normative tensions was a conflict between, on the one hand, the new authorities and protocols of the state of emergency and, on the other hand, established public authorities, connections, and bureaucratic channels. Navigating this disjuncture was a key characteristic of living through the emergency, which came to the fore when confronted with the demands of pressing obligations, such as those surrounding death. The continuity of social life through the performance of ongoing practices in negotiation with familiar authorities, social networks, and temporal expectations had to be reconciled with the dangers of the Ebola virus and the novel regulations and structures of the state of emergency.

However, the challenges that were faced by Marie's and Rachel's mourners were not entirely unfamiliar. Securing good death is never straightforward in Freetown's unpredictable environment, where flexibility in the performance of ritual is often a necessity. By virtue of the close-knit nature of family and community life, not to mention widespread material scarcity and lack of adequate medical facilities, death is always close at hand regardless of whether an unusual epidemic such as Ebola is at large. Tensions, conflict, and controversy are often present at funerals, along with the recognition that things might not go according to plan.

This chapter, building on earlier chapters, has emphasized how deep histories of crisis are prone to coming to the fore when an emergency hits. But it has also emphasized that the texture and character of day-to-day life and death immediately preceding an emergency must also be taken into serious account. This is particularly important, because without this perspective there is the temptation to impose crude models and narratives onto emergencies, such as seeing emergencies as complete ruptures from the dynamics of "ordinary" life or simply as more extreme versions of it. While some frameworks tend to emphasize the ways that preexisting inequalities are extended, others point to the ways that normal power relations are upended, at least temporarily. While both of these models are valid and often well-meaning, they can unintentionally deny the agency of people caught up in emergencies to make sense of it in their own terms. Such a perspective, by contrast, reveals how ruptures and continuities coexist during emergencies. This perspective does not take away from the hardships that people face in emergencies that are well beyond their control—or imposed on them from outside or above—but does acknowledge their active role in determining how to understand and negotiate the challenges that emergencies present. These themes are the springboard for the discussion in chapter 6 about how long-standing anthropological methods and theory can best attend to emergencies today.

ANTHROPOLOGY IN CRISIS

One morning I found an email from the UK Ministry of Defense in my inbox. A staff sergeant was asking my advice on cultural considerations around sickness and death in Sierra Leone for an initiative to establish temporary hospital facilities for Ebola patients. The email stood out to me like a sore thumb. At the time, in 2014, I was a PhD student in my midtwenties, and most of the emails I received were exchanges with my friends, family, and supervisors. I was uncertain of the implications of the email and unsure how best to respond, if at all. Was it good that the advice of an anthropologist (in training) was being sought directly by intervening forces? Did the emergency justify an email out of the blue rather than a more formal or methodical process? How much of the necessary nuance around social and cultural life in Sierra Leone could I convey in this format? Was this an opportunity to meaningfully influence global health policy for the better, or did it amount to neocolonial collusion?

In this chapter, I describe how I navigated an unexpected emergency in the course of a long-term ethnographic research project and outline some of the key lessons I learned along the way. I highlight what I consider to be three core tenets of the anthropological method, which were key in producing this book: flexibility, personal relationships, and theory from the home. During emergencies it is common for anthropological research methods to be compromised in favor of rapid policy-oriented research. While this demand is understandable, and indeed I consider flexibility to be a central asset of the anthropological method, this chapter makes the case for not abandoning what anthropologists—and social scientists employing socially embedded methods—can uniquely bring to the table.[1] My aim in this chapter is to usefully make this case to readers who are not anthropologists while also providing some practical insights from my personal experiences for anthropologists and students faced with questions and conditions similar to those that I faced during Ebola.

A considerable number of anthropologists were consulted officially during the Ebola epidemic by international actors. Several leading organizations, such as the United Nations, the World Health Organization, and the US-based Centers for Disease Control and Prevention, hired field anthropologists to assist with their work on the ground. Other primarily academic anthropologists with regional and thematic expertise banded together to form the Ebola Anthropology Response Platform and the Ebola Anthropology Initiative. These networks provided agencies and authorities with relevant anthropological insights and information about the social and cultural context in the affected countries, largely through collaboratively produced briefings on a number of different themes. I contributed to briefings on burial practices, livelihood strategies, the mobilization of youths into the response, and the underreporting of cases. Most of these topics were or ended up becoming major research interests of mine.

In my contributions to the briefings, I aimed to forward the concerns and priorities of my friends and neighbors in Freetown and also offered insights that I had learned firsthand. I hoped that this might mitigate some of the more heavy-handed aspects of the international intervention, identifying ways that could help it better meet ordinary people's needs and expectations. However, I felt uneasy about the requirements for the briefings to be only a few pages long. I understood that the short format made material more digestible than longer-form work and therefore perhaps more likely to be taken up by decision makers. But reducing complex social and cultural material to a series of bullet points was a big ask. There seemed to be an unspoken assumption that culture and social beliefs and practices (which we as anthropologists were in effect deemed experts in) were possessed only by ordinary Africans and not by intervening agencies, which were implicitly neutral and objective. If beliefs and practices could be documented in briefings, then it seemed to be assumed that these were static, unchanging things that could be basically known. This felt to be at odds with the remarkable capacities for adaption and change that I had been observing in my neighborhood, detailed in this book. Were the beliefs and practices of Freetown residents supposed to be those found during normal times (whatever that means), or were they those at play during an epidemic emergency? If the latter, could these really be separated from the impact of the international intervention and the conditions of the state of emergency?

Such concerns have long accompanied anthropological engagement. Unsurprisingly, opinions and approaches on the matter differ. Some anthropologists see public engagement as an ethical duty and lament that anthropology has lost its public relevance when compared to, say, economics. The discipline's involvement during Ebola was welcomed as a sign of relevance.[2] However, academic anthropology has historically looked down on engaged or applied anthropology as compromising the discipline's core scientific tenets by, for example, employing rapid and purpose-driven data collection rather than open-ended fieldwork. Other criticisms of engaged anthropology come from a political standpoint. Should anthropologists work uncritically within dominant power structures, just as colonial anthropologists did in the past centuries? Militant, anarchist, and decolonial anthropologies have been proposed as alternatives.[3]

My experiences of policy-oriented engagement during the 2014–2016 Ebola epidemic taught me that in an emergency when there is a felt sense of urgency, opportunity, and desire to help, core disciplinary values are too easily compromised. In the sections that follow, I outline my personal reflections on three deep-rooted tenets of the anthropological method that have closely informed the research and thinking behind this book. I believe that these elements are particularly important when doing research on or in a crisis, and I emphasize their continued importance as the discipline moves forward.

Participant Observation (It's Personal)

The first time I did anthropological fieldwork was for my undergraduate dissertation on hip-hop and kinship in New York City. I spent one month over the summer in the city, where I stayed with my grandmother. I attended concerts and block parties; interviewed rappers, artists, and educators; and spent time with my family. Earlier in the year, my department organized an information session on dissertations for students that was led by a senior professor at the time. I told him that I was planning to do fieldwork and wondered if he had any advice. He told me that conducting fieldwork takes years and that the relationships developed through it must be maintained for life. This was a rather dispiriting answer for an undergraduate with only a summer vacation available, but I was encouraged by others to go ahead with my plans.

Was it real fieldwork? Yes and no. Perhaps it would have qualified if the topic had been the dining practices of elderly Jews living on the Upper East Side. But I was not, sadly, interviewing my grandmother, who has since passed away. I learned a lot about hip-hop over my stay, but it was brief, and relationships did not last. Now that I have undertaken real fieldwork according to the senior professor's standards, I am more sympathetic to his response to my question, however discouraging it felt at the time. Anthropological, or ethnographic, fieldwork is all about personal relationships, which take time to build and nurture.

The fieldwork for this book took place over a total of two years during which I resided in an urban neighborhood in Freetown. My first visit was in 2011, and my most recent visit (at the time of writing) was in 2019. The bulk of my fieldwork was over two long stretches: almost a year between 2013 and 2014 and half a year in 2015. I was hosted by two families in the neighborhood throughout these periods. My approach was traditionally ethnographic, with at its core participant observation, the methodology developed by Bronislaw Malinowski (who founded the department at the London School of Economics where I did my PhD studies). Because I was in a city, my fieldwork was not quite the classic bounded field site of traditional ethnography, but the neighborhood gave the research a defined locus and a semidefined boundary. What became a focus of the research—family and neighborhood life among young people—was thoroughly entangled with my own experience of becoming a friend, a neighbor, and an adopted family member there.

Turning points are a common motif in fieldwork narratives. Ethnographies and reflexive accounts of the process of fieldwork itself frequently emphasize its messy and contingent character. The story goes that the anthropologist spends a long time figuring out what is going on, learning a new language and sets of social and cultural norms, amid a lot of misunderstandings and errors. And then one day something clicks. Patterns and routines start emerging, connections are made, and things begin making sense. This rarely lasts long until disruptions and the unexpected take over once again. In practice, turning points can be monthly or even weekly or daily occurrences. Sometimes there are several turning points in a single conversation. The movement between islands of clarity and oceans of unknown is an essential and fascinating part of the dynamic process of fieldwork.

But some turning points turn out to be major turning points, which, on reflection, do really represent lasting shifts in direction and gear. The first of these for me happened two or three months after I arrived in 2013 for a planned year and a half of fieldwork for my PhD research. My project at the time was a study of taxi driving and informal economies in Freetown. These themes never fully disappeared from my research (see chapter 2), but the orientation and approach radically changed. In the early months, I saw fieldwork as something I had to go out and do. Fieldwork, it felt, began once I had left the home (Foday's room and parlor) and was hanging out with drivers in the streets. This notion of fieldwork was comforting on some level because it seemed clearly defined and productive, almost like a job.

Foday and his brother Alhassan were themselves both taxi drivers. My own brother, Jacob, who lived in Freetown between 2009 and 2011, was close with Foday and Alhassan's father, James, also a driver at the time, who had introduced Jacob to his children. When I arrived in Freetown, Alhassan offered to teach me to drive. Learning to drive for the first time in an old Nissan Sunny taxi on the city's jam-packed streets was quite an initiation. After I got my license, a master class in navigating the bureaucracy of the Road Transport Authority, Alhassan would sometimes ask me to pick up private customers for him when he was busy with something else. He taught me a lot about driving, cars, traffic police, and the ins and outs of the taxi business. But the journey was more important than the destination. Along the way, I got to know Alhassan's friends, sexual partners, and family members. A number of these people lived close to where I was staying, and so gradually these relationships turned into a network, or community, of people that I was becoming part of.

At the same time, I was building relationships in and around Foday's home. Increasingly, my daily activities mapped onto established patterns of sociality. Rather than going out to do research, the process became more organic. I would share meals and watch TV with friends, stop by neighbors' houses to catch up, or receive visitors at home. Those I knew well would invite me to their family events, such as weddings, burials, and baby naming ceremonies. Sometimes I would tag along on outings around town or, on several occasions, to far-flung parts of the country on trips that would last for days or weeks.

I recorded what I observed, was told, and thought and felt into field notes, a document on my laptop with subheadings for each date. Sometimes the events of the day, such as an important family meeting, seemed like the most pressing material. But the subplots and exchanges that happened around these events were often more revealing. I aimed to write directly onto my computer, battery life permitting, when I got home. Or I would find time the following day in the early morning or during the lull in the afternoon when people take naps before children come home from school and the evening's activities commence. I would find a corner of the room where I could be alone with my recollections and notes. Or I would walk to the junction and take a shared taxi to a Lebanese café not far along the main road, where I could plug in my computer and write. Writing field notes was a regular reminder that I was an anthropologist who had come to Sierra Leone to undertake research, a fact that I found fairly easy to forget as I immersed myself in the full-time job of being a resident in a close-knit neighborhood of Freetown.

My first major turning point taught me that fieldwork is personal. It is about being in relationship with others and, as cheesy as it might sound, being in relationship with yourself. Developing and maintaining a multiplicity of interconnected relationships is key. Being exposed to many viewpoints on events as they unfold in real time reveals a layered and dynamic vision of social life and culture, compared to what can be learned through individual testimony after the fact. Relationships are never static, and viewpoints are always liable to shift. Being personally implicated in these relationships as a researcher is an important part of the equation. Going through the emotional journey with others allows you to more fully and deeply understand what is going on. But being personally implicated also means cultivating an internal touchstone necessary for building ethical and meaningful relationships. For fieldwork to be personal ultimately means going beyond any conceptual notion of personhood (even those that you encounter in fieldwork) into the realm of embodied experience, that which is felt but cannot easily be defined. Being in this kind of emotionally vulnerable relationship with others is never easy and can be especially challenging in a new place.

I regularly felt a sense of losing myself during fieldwork, which is perhaps an inevitable part of becoming socialized somewhere new. I experienced this particularly strongly when I felt that I was lacking personal space. For the nine months that Foday was hosting me we slept in the same bed, which was a common practice for friends and housemates in Freetown. And sometimes three of us shared the bed if there were guests staying over. It would get hot and uncomfortable at night, and the electricity would regularly cut off, meaning that the fan would stop working. Being dependent on my hosts and at the mercy of the unreliable National Power Authority felt to me like significant losses of the personal agency that I was accustomed to. And yet, I would feel guilty for feeling hard done by; after all, this is what I had chosen, while those around me had not chosen such material discomforts. When I moved to the Bangura family compound I had a bed to myself, but my feelings of restricted agency would persist. There was almost always loud noise, day and night. The dawn chorus began with roosters crowing and then, as the residents awoke, continued with washing, banging mortars, preparing food, greetings, and the sharing of jokes or news. In the evenings there was the hum of action films that one neighbor enjoyed watching on a television hooked up to a large stereo, a *palava* (dramatic dispute) between neighbors or family members playing out in the alleyway, or the singing of prayers and gospel songs through the night. I could expect my friends and neighbors to pay me a visit at any time. I felt a strong, palpable, sense of being socially and emotionally entangled with those around me. During one period of particularly heavy conflict in the compound, which included allegations of witchcraft, I remember being able to breathe the tension in the air.

The flip side of the discomfort that I felt around limited personal space and agency was the genuine nourishment and joy of interconnection with others. This was a striking contrast to my daily existence in London. There, I did not know my neighbors well and, arguably as a symptom of a society enmeshed in late capitalism, experienced a more lonely, individuated sense of self on a day-to-day basis. In Freetown, I felt a more contingent sense of self in which during the course of the daily routine more seemed to be at stake.

Honoring the reciprocities of social life kept me busy. Anthropologists inevitably receive a great deal in fieldwork: routine acts of hospitality and the sharing of things, time, and the intimate details of life. Sometimes building reciprocal relationships means sharing in kind, where possible, and in other cases it means contributing what is asked from you that you can uniquely provide. Sometimes, for example, I helped out with work around the house or assisted my hosts and their children with schoolwork and job applications. I was often asked to contribute to routine expenses, such as school fees, food costs, and medical expenses, as well as assist with the costs of family events such as birthday parties and funerals.

Responding to others' expectations, demands, and requests respectfully and appropriately was not always straightforward. Sometimes the expectations were unmeetable. In other cases even if I could have met them, I felt that the integrity of the research would be jeopardized if I did. There is a fine line between receiving information from others freely, on the basis of reciprocal and appropriate relationships, versus coercively, on the basis of unresolvable indebtedness. There is no easy solution to this problem. Extracting data in the absence of personal relationship, even if verbal and written consent has been received, is not only, almost by definition, unethical but is also likely to be unreliable. And yet, relationships burdened with indebtedness and obligation can also present serious issues around ethics and reliability.

Figuring out what was reasonable in terms of reciprocating was a complex calculation because it was not always clear which standards to go by. They could not simply be my own standards as an outsider. This would amount to foreign imposition, which anthropologists are carefully trained to avoid. Yet, it also felt inappropriate to adopt the standards expected of an ordinary Sierra Leonean resident of or visitor to the neighborhood, which I clearly was not. I felt that I needed standards that were somewhere in between. Part of the solution for me was shifting somewhat from a transactional vision of ethical relationships to an ethics based on being a part of a wider moral economy. In other words, I tried to be a good person in the community rather than obsessing over what I did or did not owe individuals. In practice, I nonetheless fluctuated between conflicting positionalities. Sometimes I inhabited the role of "Molay Conteh," the country name given to me, endearingly and lightheartedly, by friends and families. Or I lived up to the terms "uncle," "brother," and "son." But in the end I was Jonah Lipton, the visiting White anthropologist.

Underpinning these issues is a deeper problem of privilege and power. Regardless of how real my life in the neighborhood was, I was there by choice with a professional motive that went beyond just living there. Being White, educated, male, and materially secure were all factors that allowed me to enter into this unfamiliar space voluntarily. For LGBTI people, women, and nonbinary researchers, the risks attached to becoming immersed in a field site can be significantly greater, while building trusting relationships can be harder, whereas for non-White researchers and those doing research in or proximate to their own communities, there are inevitably different sets of demands and challenges.[4] As a White researcher coming from Britain, Sierra Leone's former colonizer, I was by default favorably placed in a racialized hierarchy that lives on from colonial times. However much anthropologists are immersed in their research sites, power differentials in the act of research itself, almost certainly compounded by other inequalities, remain.

These issues of privilege and power in ethnographic research harken back to the discipline's colonial roots. Since its inception, anthropology has specialized in the study of non-Western cultures and societies as opposed to sociology, whose remit is developed Western society. Anthropologists inevitably worked, to varying degrees, within colonial administrative structures, which gave them access to field sites and in many cases funding and employment. It is important to acknowledge that a number of anthropologists questioned and resisted coloniality through either political activities or recording empirical material and developing analytical frameworks that unsettled Eurocentric understandings of the world. But the very fact that most anthropologists from universities in the Global North continue to do fieldwork in the Global South and with marginal groups is clearly a colonial legacy in itself.[5] Understandably, some argue that the discipline can no longer be justified in its current form.[6]

It is likely that much reimagining of anthropology will take place in the coming years and decades. For the discipline to deeply address its colonial legacies, structural, material, and institutional transformations are required not only within academic institutions but also in the world at large. I see this work as largely political and collective in nature. However, I also see the personal aspect as central to this process. As I have outlined, the personal sits at the core of the practice of ethnographic fieldwork. But it is also the primary terrain where lived, embodied, transformation takes place. My emphasis on the personal is certainly not to undermine or obscure the political. Rather I see the personal in the practice of anthropology as being both closely informed by and informing broader collective politics. Such an orientation entails that we expand our understandings of what the personal and politics can look like. In good anthropological fashion, we bring a range of concepts and lived realities into critical dialogue with dominant Western understandings of these terms. However, being personal, this must not start and end as an intellectual exercise but must also be lived and practiced.

Flexibility (On Being at the Wrong Place at the Right Time)

If the first major turning point in my fieldwork was, at least in part, an internal reorientation to the fieldwork process, then the second major turning point was external: the unforeseen onset of a global health emergency. It did not happen all at once, of course. First there were rumors and reports of Ebola. Then there was the spread of the virus from Guinea to rural Sierra Leone and then from country to towns. Finally, there was the declaration of a state of emergency and large-scale humanitarian and public health intervention.

The unfolding emergency undoubtedly intensified some of the challenges of fieldwork. During the earlier stages of the epidemic, I experienced a profound disconnect between my day-to-day life and the emergency at large. For a long time I did not know anyone who had caught Ebola, which was significant from a safety point of view, as the virus was transmitted through close bodily contact. As should be clear at this point, life in the neighborhood went on amid a host of state of emergency regulations. But Ebola loomed large. All major international news platforms were reporting on it. Commercial airlines began suspending their services to the region. My girlfriend at the time had come to stay with me for a month during the summer and had difficulties getting back to London when her flight was canceled. Because the future looked uncertain and potentially dangerous, I had a decision to make as to whether to continue or interrupt my fieldwork.

In the end with some guidance from my supervisors and my department, I left Freetown until it seemed safe to return. It was not an easy decision to make. My immediate instinct based on my day-to-day life was telling me to stay, but the wider narratives at the time were telling me to leave. Some traumatic emotional material from my own family history surfaced around that time. My father's parents were both the only members of their respective families to survive the Holocaust. They left Germany as teenagers in the late 1930s, but their parents did not. Their parents were unable to get visas and hoped that the situation would not get so bad before it improved. It did not, of course, and they were unable to leave the country. I think that the hardest part of my decision to leave Freetown, however, was coming to face with an uncomfortable truth that however connected I felt to those around me, I was ultimately free to come and go pretty much as I pleased. Eventually, in any case, I would leave. My friends and host families in the Congo Town neighborhood encouraged me to go, given that it was possible. Ebola, as with many other epidemics before and since, served to highlight that while everyone is at risk in theory, in practice some are more at risk than others.

Back in London I stayed with friends in Streatham, who generously offered to host me for an indefinite period, which turned out to be five months. During this period, I became involved in the work of the Ebola Anthropology Response Platform and the Ebola Anthropology Initiative, and my PhD studies were put on hold. I was eager to get back to Freetown. I kept in close touch with my friends and contacts in the neighborhood through regular calls and exchanges of messages as well as participation in shared WhatsApp groups. And I stayed on top of the official data on Ebola cases and their whereabouts. With assistance from the Health and Safety Department at the London School of Economics, which helped me assess the risks of returning to Freetown and to devise safety and contingency plans, I returned for a further six months of fieldwork. The state of emergency was still in full effect (and would be for a year and a half longer), but it was clear that being in Freetown at this point was manageable and safe.

My second major turning point taught me the importance of flexibility in fieldwork. Flexibility is necessary in anthropological research because life, whether we like it or not, is inherently unstable and changing. Social relationships move between stability and strain. In dangerous field sites, flexibility is an essential factor in making research as safe as possible for anthropologists and interlocutors alike, which sometimes means going against narrowly formulated professional codes of ethics.[7] But flexibility also means recognizing how so-called obstacles to research can present unanticipated openings for digging deeper. Paul Rabinow in his book *Reflection on Fieldwork in Morocco* puts it like this:

> Interruptions and eruptions mock the field-worker and his inquiry; more accurately, they may be said to inform his inquiry, to be an essential part of it. The constant breakdown, it seems to me, is not just an annoying accident but a core aspect of this type of inquiry. Later I became increasingly aware that these ruptures of communication were highly revealing, and often provide to be turning points.[8]

Fieldwork must find the right balance between predetermined structure and openness to change and adjustment. We prepare by arriving with particular questions and with methodologies to answer these questions, along with a review of ethical considerations. But in the moment of doing the research itself, we must be fully responsive to what is happening there and then. Circumstances inevitably change during the course of the fieldwork, which is initially a forward-looking research agenda in which predictability is impossible. Compounded with this, research agendas are typically concocted away from the field site itself, and on arriving in the field site we might well discover that many of the assumptions we held in advance do not hold water. Or perhaps we find other questions or areas that seem more pressing or significant.

For fieldworkers, patience, care, and open-mindedness become practical approaches that are needed to create the flexibility required to be in the right place at the right time or, better perhaps, the wrong place at the right time. Events take shape in ways that are hard to predict, especially for an outsider not well attuned to the rhythms and patterns of social life. I discovered this when I showed up at weddings at the time stated on the invitation and found that the proceedings started four or five hours later. Sometimes mistakes can lead to unexpected insights, such as observing informal behind-the-scenes activities and conversations that reveal as much as the formal proceedings.[9] For me, the Ebola emergency was a macroversion of this same phenomenon, although I certainly did not always realize this at the time.

On my return to Freetown, it was clear that my research was going to have to speak to the emergency that had enveloped the field site. At the same time, I also had to prioritize staying safe. During this period, I refrained from all body contact and in particular avoided close proximity to those who were unwell. I carried around hand sanitizer, which I applied constantly. I washed my home regularly with chlorinated water and was careful about what foods I ate. I was not ready to totally abandon the questions I had been pursuing the previous year nor, more importantly, the relationships that I developed. The solution for me was to reconceptualize my fieldwork as two research projects.

The first and primary project continued from where I had left off. The focal point remained the households and networks of friends and families in which I circulated in the neighborhood. Keeping up with these relationships and routines allowed for an authentic perspective on the impact of a global health emergency on an ordinary urban community without too much probing. As it turned out, sometimes the ways that "Ebola"—the broader crisis that surrounded the epidemic—was absent from life revealed as much as where it was overt and unavoidable. At the same time, the emergency entailed unusual clarity and reflexivity about many aspects of ordinary life that were opaque or taken for granted beforehand. It was almost as if everyone had become an anthropologist during the epidemic, expounding their own analyses and theories of culture and society.

The second research project, which really started as a smaller side project, involved a more probing and active approach. I wanted to identify a direct and unambiguous viewpoint on the emergency but one that connected to the social world that I already knew in Freetown. This project became my fieldwork with the official Ebola burial teams. One of my primary interlocutors and friends—Peter, the motorbike taxi rider—was enrolled in the official Ebola response as a bike rider attached to a burial team, as described in chapter 2. He invited me to meet the team. After gaining permission from the team leader, I met up with the team once a day every week or two and spent the day with them. The burial teams were well trained and equipped, and as such I was not at great risk of contagion. I took additional precautions, such as keeping my distance when they were physically handling a body and from the families they interacted with.

Burials were a definitive interface between families and state of emergency authorities and protocols, revealing critical dynamics in the ways that ordinary people made sense of and responded to the emergency. Although it was a new focus, this attention to burials nevertheless dovetailed closely with my established focuses and primary research project. The members of the burial teams, mostly young men who were trained to perform family funerary rituals, represented a continuity of my interest in the intersections of informal economies, youth, and family. At the same time, following several deaths in my community including in the compound I was living in (see chapter 5) and observing attitudes and approaches to burial from that vantage point, the material I was getting from my time with the team became part of a more complete picture.

The interplay of events and crises, whether micro or macro, sudden or drawn out, gets to the heart of the methodology of this book. Microevents form much of the ethnographic material: burials, a pregnancy and a baby naming ceremony, disputes at home and at work, meetings, accidents, and lockdowns. Looming above these was the macroevent of a global health emergency. The microevents presented in this book are not only useful narrative devices through which to illustrate to the reader what social life in Freetown looks like but are also in themselves focal points for protagonists and participants around which social life is scrutinized and analyzed. It was around these events that the wider event of Ebola often became most tangible and real. Combining my two projects revealed two forms of crisis that came together during Ebola: a temporary health emergency and an ongoing crisis of social reproduction connected to a long-unfolding political and economic crisis.

My approach to fieldwork and analysis in this book follows on from some of the innovations of Max Gluckman and his colleagues in the early and mid-twentieth century, who became known as the Manchester School. Contrary to structural-functionalists orthodoxy at the time, the Manchester School set out not to discover singular, static social orders in their respective societies of research but instead to document and understand change. Working through the Rhodes-Livingstone Institute, many examined industrialization, urbanization, and colonialism in southern Africa, often through a politically critical lens. At the cornerstone of their methodology was the "extended-case study method," also known as "situational analysis." Through rich ethnographic recording of the event, insight into transformative social processes was gained.[10]

The extended-case method did not see crisis, or emergency, as an obstacle to the investigation of ordinary social life but instead saw windows into it. During the event or situation, a bigger picture of the macroforces governing society is revealed to both participants and anthropologists alike. Bruce Kapferer summarizes it like this: "a major point that Gluckman stresses is that it is in crisis—in the situation as crisis and specifically in events that constitute concentrated and intense dimensions of the overall crisis of the situation—that the vital forces and principles already engaged in social action (or taking form in the event itself) are both revealed and rendered available to anthropological analysis."[11] While eventful times such as emergencies can present particular challenges to knowledge production—with potential difficulties in access, greater risks, breakdowns in trust, and information vacuums—they also present unique potential for understanding social agency and change when transformation is inevitable.[12] During global health crises, when the pressures for anthropologists to respond directly to narrow health problems are amplified, maintaining ethnographic reflexivity and openness are particularly valuable.[13]

Theory from the Home

The global reach of the COVID-19 pandemic resulted in large swaths of the global population experiencing the daily realities of life in a health emergency firsthand. Many of us sustained months of lockdown, with restrictions on work, travel, and social life. Our experiences were, of course, far from uniform. As epidemics tend to reveal rather starkly, some people are more vulnerable than others. In many instances preexisting inequalities—such as the quality of health care, housing, type of work, and hierarchies of class, gender, age, and race—are reproduced in the form of differential risk.[14] Some people are more able to retreat into safety than others. However, it is safe to say that for many people of many different backgrounds and locations, the COVID-19 pandemic entailed significant amounts of time spent at home and greater interdependence among family and other domestic relations.

At the same time, many of us were glued to the news cycle and social media feeds, where we followed the dramas of governments and public institutions as they went about enacting often unpopular public health measures. Catching up with friends and family at the time, I noticed a disconnect between what we talked about and the reality of our day-to-day lives. What dominated conversations was the public face of the crisis: the political dramas, the rate of new cases and deaths, comparing responses in different places, and speculating about when things might ease up or go back to normal. Sometimes we talked about personal stories, such as people we knew or friends of friends who caught the virus. We criticized others for not taking precautions seriously enough. But we did not, at least in my fairly diverse circle, seem to have the language or the tendency to talk about the pandemic emergency as a domestic experience even though this was the arena that most directly defined our social experiences of it.

It is not coincidental that during health emergencies such as COVID-19 and Ebola, which are conceptualized as "public," the dominant discourse tends to marginalize ordinary, domestic, personal, and private concerns. Maintaining the integrity of the government, the economy, and the state—and in more masked ways the interests of social networks we might refer to as the ruling class—is often prioritized over the maintenance and long-term priorities of ordinary families and other domestic and intimate relationships. The prioritization of "public" during epidemics and other emergencies is particularly pronounced but is in keeping with long-standing trends in Western political thought. When talking about "politics" today, most people expect a conversation about governments, parliaments, and politicians. These are traditionally male domains, associated with the governance of the nation-state. This is why the second-wave feminist slogan "the personal is political" is radical and enduring (albeit easily co-opted for individualistic and consumerist purposes). The widespread coding of the home and the domestic as female spaces undoubtedly contributes to their being deemed secondary.

I am not saying that demands on the state and other public bodies should not be made in times of emergency. During epidemics, political organizing and collective pressure can be critical to ensuring fairer and more effective responses. And whether we like it or not, most of us do live, at least in part, within the governance structures of a nation-state. But the point here is that this is only one side of the story. The other side begins at home but expands beyond to a broader vision of society at large. From this perspective, the home is not taken for granted, parochial, or fixed in its ways but instead is dynamic, changing, and far-reaching. Epidemics such as Ebola and COVID-19 should make this clear to us all even if we lack the language to talk about it.

Anthropology has much to offer to this side of the story, because it has long been its specialty. Over more than a century of ethnographic research, the home and the family have been at the epicenter of the discipline. With the early (and arguably enduring) pigeonholing of anthropology as the study of non-Western small-scale societies, its archetypal subjects are nomadic hunter-gatherers, pastoralists, and remote farming and fishing communities. In such face-to-face communities in the absence of (or, more realistically, on the fringes of) the state and the industrial economy, family and home are at the heart of social, political, and economic life. Given this, it is almost an anthropological truism to state that the social, political, and economic cannot be understood as distinct categories, as they are purported to be in modern Western frameworks. Kinship theory, which emphasized the interconnection of these domains, was for many decades the principal preoccupation of the discipline, particularly in the British and French anthropological traditions.

The practice of ethnographic fieldwork also favors situating the home as a starting place for theory. During fieldwork, many anthropologists, including myself, are hosted by people who in turn become their primary interlocutors and research subjects. When anthropologists are not hosted by interlocutors, the processes of making and visiting homes still tend to be instructive parts of being socialized into a new place. The quotidian and personal aspects of the ethnographic method make it particularly suited to the study of ordinary life. As anthropology turned its attention to urban and Western settings—alongside engagement with theoretical frameworks from sociology, geography, political theory, and cultural studies—the discipline's orientation toward day-to-day sociality has remained intact. The study of kinship has become less prevalent in recent decades partly in the aftermath of David Schneider's influential critique that the concept is itself Eurocentric.[15] However, in widely disparate contemporary global settings, family continues to be hugely significant in structuring social life. As Adam Kuper recently put it, "The situation of kinship studies is paradoxical. Wherever we ethnographers go, we find that most people live in family households, obsess over marriage choices, celebrate kinship rituals, and quarrel over inheritance. And yet remarkably few anthropologists are writing about this sort of thing."[16]

Perhaps the global spread of family makes it particularly prone to accommodating our unexamined notions and assumptions. It is easy to impose one's own understandings of family into a context in which family might superficially look somewhat similar but actually represents and amount to something quite different. And there is the tendency to taint the family of the Other with unexamined (or examined) prejudices, for example, labeling non-White families as broken. Both of these patterns are common during public health interventions. Even sympathetic programs, such as psychosocial support, can inadvertently impose Western psychological constructs onto contexts where they do not readily apply.[17] During Ebola, international actors routinely blamed family practices of burial and care for the severity of the epidemic. Behind this was a blurred vision of local culture as static and backward rather than adaptable and contingent.

It is easy to hold prejudices about that which you know little. Unlike the public sphere, which is—almost by definition—widely visible, the spaces of family and home are not. Trust and time are required for outsiders to begin to under-stand them. Unlike public institutions, family is not open for business or in ses-sion at a particular time but instead operates around the clock, often in quite coded and opaque ways. As many anthropologists, myself included, find out dur-ing fieldwork, accessing domestic and family spaces pretty much requires that you become family first. This must be learned through observation, instruction, and practice. Fully and personally participating in life in and around the home is not just a means for recording rich ethnographic material, such as the unfold-ing of family dramas, intimate revelations, and unusual ritual practices. The vast majority of what we encounter and experience does not make it beyond field notes but does allow us to gain a felt firsthand appreciation of the rhythms and contours of ordinary life. And in the process, meaningful, complex, and (hope-fully) caring relationships are formed. This becomes the starting point for a different vision of society and crisis to emerge.

In this chapter, I have focused on three interconnected areas of anthropological research that are at once deep-rooted in the discipline's history and hold renewed value in the study of and engagement in crises today: the personal, flexibility, and theory from the home. Their value lies in part in the fact that other disci-plines and actors often do not attend to or practice them and in many cases do not have the language or method to do so. Yet, these are areas that anthropologists are liable to discard or compromise in the event of a pressing emergency when, ironically, these are the times when they matter most. As I have emphasized here, these are not tenets to be blindly adhered to. Rather, they center around the lived, intimate, embodied, contingent, and shifting practice of fieldwork and call for open-ended and open-hearted attention to the practice itself.

As such, I cannot prescribe what embracing these elements of the anthropo-logical method will look like for others. For myself, they entailed gaining first-hand experience of ways that global histories and political and economic forces structure the most intimate of relationships. It meant going through uncomfort-able and unsettling experiences during fieldwork, including adapting to novel constraints on my agency, navigating new dangers, and confronting aspects of myself, particularly my privilege, that was more convenient to ignore. It meant being implicated in other people's projects and struggles on their terms and learning, however imperfectly, how to build caring relationships across the fault lines of social conditioning and inequalities. Although I went on to tell the story of this book, I have come to recognize that this book is only one of many stories and incalculable outcomes from the process of research that it has come out of.

CONCLUSION

It was mid-2020, and I was catching up with James Bangura on WhatsApp. COVID-19 had become global. Reconnecting with my friends in Freetown at that time was both strange and comforting for me. There was a surreal sense of déjà vu. What we were going through and the ways we talked about it were remarkably reminiscent of Ebola, less than five years earlier. These conversations reminded me that while such epidemic emergencies can feel endless when case numbers do not seem to be going down, eventually they can come to some form of end. After some back-and-forth with James on more general aspects of the pandemic and the government's response to it, he told me that his wife Aisha was pregnant again. "This time in corona, first time was Ebola," he wrote, referring to the tumultuous birth of their firstborn child, described in chapter 5.

In 2019 I spent four months in Freetown. I stayed with James and Aisha in their family compound, as I had done during my fieldwork between 2013 and 2015 during Ebola. It was now two years since the Ebola state of emergency was officially lifted. James and Aisha had moved into the room that I had stayed in before, while I now slept in the former room of James's stepmother Leah, who left the compound after her husband's passing in 2016. It was strange being back. It felt like a lot had changed but, at the same time, that things were almost exactly as they were. In the compound, James was grappling with the responsibilities he had taken on after his father's death. He was expected to look after a group of younger cousins and siblings who were now crowded into the other rooms of the house. There was a national election earlier in the year in which the main opposition party had come into power. One evening the neighborhood was saturated by the roar of the crowd at the national stadium, across the valley, during a game between old rivals, the East End Lions and the Mighty Blackpool. This was the first official league game since the Sierra Leone Premiere League had shut down during the Ebola state of emergency almost five years earlier.

In 2019 I felt more grown-up than the young man who first stepped foot in the Congo Town neighborhood in Freetown in 2011. But it was something akin to a younger version of me that I was forced to reinhabit while back, the version of me that most people seemed to remember. The daily rhythms of neighborhood life—with all its richness of sociality—and the kinds of challenges that its residents were facing were familiar from my previous visits: financial hardship and its knock-on effects, disputes with neighbors and within households, and untreated illness leading to premature death. The city's formal medical infrastructure was still poorly equipped to serve a population of its size. Little of the infrastructure that was introduced to the country during Ebola had been effectively converted to serve the routine health needs of its population, in large part because it was not built to do so.

This fact was really brought home to me during a workshop that I participated in at Njala University in Sierra Leone with colleagues from the London School of Economics. One afternoon we visited a former Ebola treatment center not far from the rural campus, where we received an informal tour by a former nurse who had worked there only a few years prior. The center was locked, inaccessible to the public, and we were struck by how little remained intact: practically just the foundations, which were now encroached by plants and trees in and around the complex (figure 5). The image of the derelict and yet still relatively

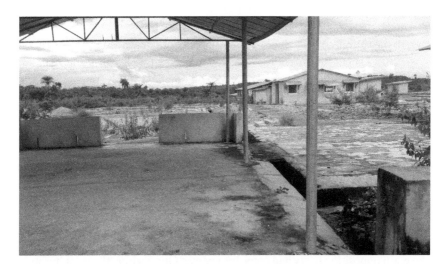

FIGURE 5.   The remnants of an Ebola treatment center.

new treatment center was like a metaphor for the short-termist and narrow priorities of the international intervention.

Even if the Ebola emergency did not fundamentally change the public health infrastructure of Sierra Leone or indeed its political, economic, and social orders, it was nonetheless significant for those who lived through it. For some people, Ebola's legacy was defined by the loss of loved ones to the disease or at the time of the outbreak. For others, such as James and Aisha, Ebola lived on in the story of their firstborn child and the reconfiguring of familial and intimate relationships that happened around that period. For others, such as members of the burial team, the emergency lasted in the opportunities that came from landing salaried work and the redundancy packages that they sought eventually coming through. Peter, the bike rider, had finished his university studies and found work as a research consultant. He told me that many of his former colleagues from the team, including Alimamy, had invested their packages in overland and overseas migration attempts to Europe, the Middle East, and elsewhere.

Starting with the "Ordinary"

This book offers an unusual perspective on a global health emergency. Rather than beginning with an extraordinary virus or disease, as most epidemic narratives do—often playing on tropes of alterity and exoticism—here we began with the ordinary. The protagonists of this story are not government officials, scientists, or international humanitarian responders but rather the residents of an ordinary neighborhood in a city that became swept up in a global emergency. On center stage here are the intimate spaces of the home and other corners of the neighborhood where its residents regularly socialize rather than hospitals and conference rooms (although these have featured too). Foregrounded are the priorities and practices of young people, with particular attention placed on familial relationships, movement through the life course, and work. These priorities tended to be expansive and long-term, in contrast with the narrower and more short-term priorities of international agencies and actors. Instead of relying on testimony after the fact, this account weaves between what was spoken and known by people in real time during the emergency and the realms of observed activity that are embodied and unspoken.

Starting with the ordinary is not just about people, priorities, practices, and places but is also about *time*. As an anthropologist, I was in an unexpected situation of finding myself embedded in a field site while a major emergency unfolded around me. This allowed for a granular perspective on what the epidemic looked like as it played out, which in turn pointed me to question established scholarly frameworks for making sense of crises. A major takeaway from this book is that emergencies are not linear events. Ebola did not introduce ambiguities and difficulties around care, intimacy, and health; rather, the Ebola emergency animated existing and deep-rooted problems. Thus, some of the uncertainties of emergencies are not necessarily the product of the emergency itself, even though this might appear to be the case, but instead are the ways that emergencies interact with what has come before. As we saw in the case of "black" and "white" systems of burials, deep-rooted historical patterns going back to the Atlantic slave trade and abolitionism were unearthed during Ebola, providing a framework that structured people's understandings and responses to it.

To add a further layer in what I have described as the extraordinary ordinary, emergencies can paradoxically allow for forms of normality that are normally absent. This was especially the case for many of the young people at the heart of this book for whom the Ebola emergency presented unusual clarity on the contradictory expectations of different overlapping social orders in which they were enmeshed. The existence of these different social orders was made unusually plain during the international intervention, manifesting as two constructed worlds, one local and undeveloped and the other global and developed. But these orders were already found in many domains of life in Freetown, such as the relational order of kinship versus the transactional order of business in and around the home, and in the registers of formal and precarious informal work on the city's streets. The clarity that came with the emergency had material implications for those we were able to broker and navigate between social orders, drawing on long-standing approaches to social mobility in Sierra Leone and other postcolonial contexts. This found expression in employment opportunities, the realigning of familial relationships, new relations between precarious workers and the state, and openings for honorable progression through the life course.

In flipping the ways that emergency narratives are normally structured, this book contains a broader message with both scholarly and political implications, namely that we must increasingly swing our focus from the extraordinary to the ordinary. The extraordinary understandably captures much of our attention by virtue of being unusual. Such a bias is particularly blatant in mainstream media and news reporting, in which shocking stories attract eyeballs and ears and, of course, advertising and sales revenue. In connected ways, the prioritization of the extraordinary dictates where budgets are directed in the spheres of public and global health, humanitarianism, and international development. For example, routine illnesses such as malaria and typhoid, while ultimately more deadly in Sierra Leone, are much less "sexy" than viruses such as Ebola and therefore receive less attention. A similar instinct pervades popular and professional culture. Academics are valued for saying something original and finding something new. Across the board, the drive to brand and market ourselves pressures us to discover what makes us unique. This moves attention away from engaging seriously and critically with the multiple layers of the ordinary, which in the end speak most closely to the reality of most people's lives.

Following the lead of the residents of the Congo Town neighborhood, it is not only that the ordinary reveals much of the lived reality of emergencies that becomes concealed in extraordinary framings and discourses but also that emergencies present surprisingly rich opportunities to cast our critical attention on different dimensions of ordinary life. By virtue of being time marked as "emergency," they reveal with unusual clarity the range of what people find to be pressing concerns for themselves and others around them and where the openings and limitations lie. In this process, the basic constructability of social, cultural, political, and economic life becomes revealed in a new light. Additionally, the disparity between the expectations that people place on themselves and each other and the material possibilities of meeting those expectations becomes particularly stark. This can lead to flexible, accelerated, and creative reworkings of conventions, as we saw in the case of family ritual at various stages along the life course and in approaches to work by young Ebola responders. Such reworkings can also lead to lasting transformations in familial relationships and perhaps to forms of politics that question the vast inequities of our global economic and political structures.

Crisis and Emergency

In this book I have set out to describe and theorize the significance of emergencies in places and among people for whom crisis has become more of a norm than an exception. The young men and women at the heart of this story fit the profile of those considered to be living amid the uncertainties and precarities of ongoing crisis today. This crisis can be described as having a public and private face (although I hope that this book has somewhat complicated this distinction). The public face is the economic and state structure that they live and work within. Young people criticize the government for not serving their material interests and, particularly informal workers, blame the police for holding them back. On a larger scale, extractive global economic arrangements ensure that only a meager percentage of Sierra Leone's wealth in natural resources benefits ordinary people, directly or indirectly. Thus, Freetown remains one of the world's poorest cities although it has a rich, cosmopolitan history and culture. Freetown, like many cities in the Global South, is overcrowded and underserviced, with communities suffering from floods, fires, and other environmental disasters on an almost annual basis. The private face of the crisis might be summed up in the complaint I regularly hear among youths in Freetown, particularly young men, that it is practically impossible to find "real love" and that there is too much "money love." This challenge extends beyond securing stable intimate partnerships and the land and resources required to build a home to the possibility of honorable progression through the entire life course from marriage and the birth of children to death.

Ebola, however, represented something more temporary and defined than this slow-burn contemporary crisis. The dangers were more clearly articulated and quantifiable even if they were scary and unusual. Yet, as we have discovered, the Ebola emergency—and indeed all epidemics—take on a range of political, economic, and, centrally here, social meanings and significances that far exceeds the contours of biomedicine and epidemiology. In part, the term "Ebola," as it was understood in Freetown, was closely connected the public health emergency of Ebola; in other words, the numerous ways that the novel disease and the public health protocols and regulations put in place to control it directly impacted people's lives. But "Ebola" was also a way of talking about and responding to the broader crisis described above in ways that were transformative for many of those involved, partly in ways that accentuated existing problems and partly in ways that proved to be unusual solutions to them. The efficacy of the time of emergency for such transformative social processes was connected to the fact that it was understood as temporary. During this period there was an unusual alignment of attention across many strata of society, including internationally, toward a shared problem, while novel material flows and bureaucracies in the public health response were not yet fully tainted with the patterns of exclusion that the marginalized are accustomed to.

Bringing It All Back Home

This book is not only an account of the Ebola emergency in Freetown, with all its specificities and peculiarities, but in keeping with the anthropological tradition, it also aims to deepen our understanding of something more global and shared. When I started writing, I was not expecting that the world would go through a pandemic before I had finished. Most readers will have had direct personal experience of some of what I have described. My experience during Ebola made me particularly attuned to the mismatch between the ways that COVID-19 was being talked about in public and private forums and people's actual day-to-day experiences of life at the time. I wondered whether people across the globe, particularly in the West, would become more sympathetic when considering the challenges of balancing ongoing commitments and routines with the demands of a public health emergency that was lacking in the widespread blaming of culture by international and local observers during Ebola. Perhaps this is wishful thinking.

This book does not just aim to promote a richer analysis of Ebola and other emergencies but also asks us to question what we take to be normal and ordinary in our own lives. In reality, we rarely encounter the stability and predictability that we might associate with these notions or indeed yearn for. This is certainly the case when considering the flux of the material world and natural phenomena but is also the case in our human social worlds too. Social reproduction and intergenerational cultural transmission, even in normal times, rely on breaks and ruptures. This is particularly overt during rituals, when social rules and hierarchies tend to shift from the sincere "as is" of the day-to-day into the subjunctive mode of "as if." The "as if," following the analysis of Victor Turner and others, might signify a world of dark fantasy emerging into view from beneath the surface or, in more mild, playful form, the temporary blurring of social boundaries and categories through embodied performance.[1] However, such dynamics are at play not only in the rituals that we overtly socially orchestrate but also in emergencies that can appear much less within our control. Emergencies are particularly powerful catalysts for both change and continuity in society, especially for those who are stuck. It does not seem coincidental that family ritual was such a focal point for young people in Freetown during Ebola. In the midst of major upheavals of one sort or another today, there is a striking persistence, if not growing importance, of family as a defining social institution in old and young people's lives, however flexible and contested this concept might be.

Emergencies, in particular epidemics, are critical occasions when we define and redefine what we value in our lives and share with others. As normal routines become disrupted (and especially if we are locked down in our homes or neighborhoods), we are forced to confront aspects of ourselves and our relationships with others that otherwise can easily be missed or go unacknowledged. This can be a highly challenging process but one that forces us to glimpse more acutely the ways that we are vitally reliant on others around us and those beyond sight. Viral epidemics reveal on one level what we fundamentally share as human beings. They spread across national borders and between bodies that bypass the social boundaries and categories that we erect between ourselves and others. And yet, emergencies are also times when we redefine and reinforce division and distinction. We see securitized policies of containment, discourses of blame, and new (and old) patterns of exclusion. If we are to better understand the deeper causes and longer-term consequences of emergencies today, we must better appreciate not only the range of experiences, priorities, and needs of people caught up in them but also what they tell us about being human.

Notes

INTRODUCTION

1. On pandemic bonds and private equity models of global health financing, see Erikson, "Global Health Futures?"

2. United Nations Development Programme, *Assessing the Socio-economic Impacts of Ebola Virus Disease in Guinea, Liberia and Sierra Leone: The Road to Recovery*, 2014, https://www.undp.org/content/dam/rba/docs/Reports/EVD%20Synthesis%20Report%2023Dec2014.pdf.

3. Seisay and Kamara, *Sierra Leone 2015: Population and Housing Census; Thematic Report on Mortality*.

4. In chapter 6, I specifically outline practical and theoretical insights that I learned from my personal experiences of navigating a long-term research project in the face of an unexpected emergency.

5. There are a number of in-depth ethnographic accounts of local responses to historic and contemporary intervention in rural Sierra Leone. See Ferme, *The Underneath of Things*; Ferme, *Out of War*; Leach, *Rainforest Relations*; Richards, *Ebola: How a People's Science Helped End an Epidemic*; and Shaw, *Memories of the Slave Trade*.

6. See Farmer, *Fever, Feuds, and Diamonds*; and Rashid, "Epidemics and Resistance in Colonial Sierra Leone during the First World War."

7. Roitman, *Anti-Crisis*, questions the usefulness of the concept of crisis, given its breadth of meaning and susceptibility to manipulation. Rather than cast the term aside, in this book I argue that crisis remains an important critical concept but that we need to better understand, both theoretically and empirically, the relationship between an ongoing crisis and a temporary emergency.

8. As Calhoun, "The Idea of Emergency," points out, "Emergency focuses attention on the immediate event, and not on its causes. It calls for a humanitarian response, not political or economic analysis. The emergency has become a basic unit of global affairs" (30).

9. Taking inspiration from Walter Benjamin, Agamben, *State of Exception*, famously argues that the ability to declare a "state of exception" rather than upholding the rule of law has become central to contemporary state sovereignty.

10. On subjectivities of crisis as an ongoing phenomenon, see Berlant, *Cruel Optimism*; Hage, "Waiting Out the Crisis"; and Mbembe and Roitman, "Figures of the Subject in Times of Crisis."

11. On waithood, see Honwana, *Youth, Waithood and Protest Movements in Africa*. For models that emphasize the difficulties for African youths in escaping their marginal status, on social navigation see Vigh, "Social Death and Violent Life Chances," and on crisis in context see Vigh, "Crisis and Chronicity." However, waithood and social navigation differ in their characterizations of structure and agency. In waithood the social and political structure in which youths are situated is rigid and static. Meaningful mobility takes place through horizontal mass collective action, such as protest movements. In social navigation, the structure—that is, the young men's social environment in a violent context—is constantly in motion and shifting. All available escape routes from marginalization entail in one way or another the joining of vertical patrimonial networks.

12. Ambiguity is a recurring theme in the anthropology of Sierra Leone. See Diggins, *Coastal Sierra Leone*; Ferme, *The Underneath of Things*; and Jackson, *Life within Limits*.

13. Anthropological research emphasizes that "youth," rather than being a universal biological age-based category, is instead a social category, as famously demonstrated in the study by Mead, *Coming of Age in Samoa*. Thus, in a given social context the biological ages of those occupying the category of youth differs. And indeed, in the same social context individuals can move in and out of the category in a nonlinear manner, as emphasized in regard to the theory of "vital-conjectures" in Johnson-Hanks, "On the Limits of Life Stages in Ethnography." As a social category, youth gains meaning through its interaction with other social categories, such as religious affiliation, gender, class, ethnicity, and race. On the crisis of youth in Africa, see, for example, Abbink and van Kessel, *Vanguard or Vandals* and Honwana and de Boeck, *Makers and Breakers*. For more recent ethnographic studies in urban settings, see Janson, *Islam, Youth and Modernity in the Gambia*; Masquelier, *Fada*; Smith, *To Be a Man Is Not a One-Day Job*; and Di Nunzio, *The Act of Living*.

14. United Nations, Department of Economic and Social Affairs, *Population Facts: Youth Population Trends and Sustainable Development*.

15. On factors leading to the youth uprisings in Sierra Leone, see Peters, *War and the Crisis of Youth in Sierra Leone*. On child soldiers in the aftermath of the war, see Shepler, *Childhood Deployed*.

16. See, for example, Banton, *West African City*; Evans-Pritchard, *The Nuer*; Fortes, *The Web of Kinship among the Tallensi*; and Meillassoux, *Maidens, Meal and Money*.

17. On youth and stuckedness in Rwanda, see Sommers, *Stuck*.

18. See, for example, the widely viewed HBO documentary *Orphans of Ebola*.

19. For work in Sierra Leone, see Parker et al., "Ebola and Public Authority"; and Richards, *Ebola: How a People's Science Helped End an Epidemic*.

20. See, for example, Farmer et al., *Reimagining Global Health*; Fassin, *When Bodies Remember*; and Hunter, *Love in the Time of Aids*.

21. On witchcraft and intimacy in West Africa, see Geschiere, *Witchcraft, Intimacy, and Trust*.

22. Reece, "'We Are Seeing Things,'" charts similar entanglements between kinship and crisis in the context of AIDS in Botswana.

23. The ordinary in crisis, particularly conflict and violence, is the focus of a number of anthropological studies in recent decades. Das, *Life and Words*, charts how major violence in India's modern history, such as partition, entered the "recesses of the ordinary" in its aftermath, playing out at the everyday, gendered, and subjective levels. In Africa, various studies have pointed to how the ordinary and related notions are prioritized by people during and after conflict. See, for example, Bolten, *I Did It to Save My Life*; Hoffman and Lubkemann, "Introduction: West-African Warscapes"; and Porter, *After Rape*. The context of an epidemic emergency has parallels to wartime but also some important differences, as outlined in chapter 4.

24. On these two different notions of normal and ordinary, see Bolten, "The Agricultural Impasse"; and Warner, *The Trouble with Normal*.

25. See Turner, *The Forest of Symbols*.

26. Turner, *The Anthropology of Performance*, 42.

27. See Seligman et al., *Ritual and Its Consequences*.

28. See Comaroff and Comaroff, *Of Revelation and Revolution*; Englund, *Prisoners of Freedom*; Ferguson, *Expectations of Modernity*; and James, *Songs of the Women Migrants*.

29. On porous social orders in contemporary anthropology, see Gershon, "Porous Social Orders." On the notion of two orders in theories of crisis, see Narotzky and Besnier, "Crisis, Value, and Hope."

30. As Gershon, "Porous Social Orders," notes, "Porous boundaries let people, ideas, objects, and forms circulate between social orders in ways that often keep distinctions between social orders durable" (405).

31. See Vaughan, *Curing Their Ills.*

32. Jane Guyer's formative study, *Marginal Gains,* shows how West Africa's long-standing entanglement with foreign markets and influences led to the emergence of a multiplicity of value scales and economic logics, from equivalence to asymmetrical exchange determined by social factors such as status. The possibility of "marginal gain" occurs at the transactional threshold between registers through "conversions."

1. MARGINALIZED COSMOPOLITANS

1. Vaughan, *Curing Their Ills.*

2. Wald, *Contagious.*

3. For more on youth performance and global interconnection in contemporary Sierra Leone, see Bolten, *Serious Youth in Sierra Leone.*

4. Fyfe, *A History of Sierra Leone,* 120.

5. The population of greater Freetown, including adjacent neighborhoods and towns in Western Area, is estimated to be two million.

6. Fortes, *Kinship and the Social Order,* defined "neighborliness" as social relations connected by spatial proximity, suffused with values of kinship. This is similar to what is more recently described by Bjarnesen and Utas, "Introduction Urban Kinship," as "urban kinship," which pays attention to the micropolitical facets of urban relatedness.

7. Cohen, *The Politics of Elite Culture.*

8. On African cities in the twenty-first century, see Nuttall and Mbembe, *Johannesburg*; Simone, *City Life from Jakarta to Dakar*; and De Boeck and Plissart, *Kinshasa.*

9. See Hoffman, *The War Machines*; and Enria, *The Politics of Work in a Post-Conflict State.*

10. On stuckedness, see Sommers, *Stuck.* On waithood, see Honwana, *Youth, Waithood and Protest Movements in Africa.*

11. See the notion of African youths as shifters in Durham, "Disappearing Youth."

12. Rodney, *A History of the Upper Guinea Coast, 1545–1800,* argued that local social transformations at this time were inextricably linked to the external trade that had interacted with coastal societies for a much longer period.

13. Stilwell, *Slavery and Slaving in African History.*

14. Lovejoy and Hogendorn, *Slow Death for Slavery.*

15. Little, *The Mende of Sierra Leone.*

16. Asiama, "Land Accessibility and Urban Agriculture in Freetown, Sierra Leone."

17. Fyfe, *A History of Sierra Leone,* 296.

18. The most recent epidemic of smallpox in Sierra Leone was in 1968–1969, which, as with Ebola, was transmitted around burial practices. See Hopkins et al., "Smallpox in Sierra Leone."

19. On the ways that nonequivalence between Black and White lives was built into the spatial organization of Ebola treatment centers, see Hirsch, "Race and the Spatialisation of Risk during the 2013–2016 West African Ebola Epidemic."

20. On the legacy of Spanish flu during Ebola and in particular the remarkable parallels and forgetting, see Farmer, "Ebola, the Spanish Flu, and the Memory of Disease." "Although Ebola responders and public-health authorities have short memories—no one, in 2014, seemed to remember that mass graves had been dug before in Kambia or Port Loko, save during the civil war that ended a dozen years earlier" (68).

21. Rashid, "Patterns of Rural Protest."

22. Cohen, *The Politics of Elite Culture.*

23. Harris, *Sierra Leone.*

24. Richards, *Fighting for the Rain Forest.*

25. On performativity of rebel combat, see Richards, *Fighting for the Rain Forest.* On post-Fordist economic practices, see Hoffman, *The War Machines.*

26. On the mixed impact of the formal peace-building process in Sierra Leone, see Mieth, "Bringing Justice and Enforcing Peace?"; Allen, *Trial Justice*, charts similar mismatches between local and international notions of justice surrounding the International Criminal Court in Uganda.

27. Polman, *The Crisis Caravan.*

28. On the exceptionality of HIV in the postwar period, see Benton, *HIV Exceptionalism.* This mirrors the privileged status of Ebola in international funding priorities during the 2014–2016 epidemic.

29. See accounts by Black, *Belly Woman*, and Walsh and Johnson, *Getting to Zero*, about their experiences of working in the international response in Sierra Leone during the Ebola epidemic.

30. As Benton notes, "In part, the difficulty of decoupling security and aid is related the 'defensiveness' embedded in the aid landscape and everyday aid practices." Benton, "Whose Security?," 27.

31. On the connections between brokerage and neoliberalism in Africa, see James, "The Return of the Broker."

2. HAZARD PAY

1. See Lazar, "A 'Kinship Anthropology of Politics'?," and Kapsea and McNamara, "'We Are Not Just a Union, We Are a Family'" on notions of labor unionism as kinship.

2. For more on the violent politics of commercial bike riding in Freetown and its connection to national political processes, see Enria, *The Politics of Work in a Post-Conflict State.*

3. For more on the history of commercial bike riding in provincial Sierra Leone and the continuities of wartime dynamics in the postwar period, see Bürge, "Riding the Narrow Tracks of Moral Life"; Menzel, "Between Ex-Combatization and Opportunities for Peace"; and Peters, "From Weapons to Wheels."

4. Bolt, *Zimbabwe's Migrants and South Africa's Border Farms*, describes how economic crises in southern Africa similarly led to new configurations of formal and informal work.

5. World Health Organization, "Ebola Response Roadmap."

6. On the coercive elements of state and foreign intervention during recent epidemics in Africa, see Abdullah and Rashid, *Understanding West Africa's Ebola Epidemic*; Chigudu, *The Political Life of an Epidemic*; and Parker et al., "Epidemics and the Military."

7. Agamben, *State of Exception.*

8. Ethnographic investigations of interventions—particularly in the world of international development—have tended to make more nuanced arguments, emphasizing how the failings of particular projects serve to nonetheless reproduce global and local hierarchies and inequalities. See Englund, *Prisoners of Freedom*; Ferguson, *The Anti-Politics Machine*; and Gardner, *Discordant Development.*

9. Farmer, *Infections and Inequalities.*

10. Richards, *Ebola.*

11. Parker et al., "Ebola and Public Authority."

12. On resistance during the 2014–2016 West African Ebola epidemic, see Fairhead, "Understanding Social Resistance to the Ebola Response in the Forest Region of the Republic of Guinea"; Marcis et al., "Three Acts of Resistance during the 2014–16 West

Africa Ebola Epidemic"; and Wilkinson and Fairhead, "Comparison of Social Resistance to Ebola Response in Sierra Leone and Guinea Suggests Explanations Lie in Political Configurations Not Culture."

13. Tapscott, *Arbitrary States*, argues that arbitrariness has become institutionalized in postcolonial African states.

14. Benton, *HIV Exceptionalism*, describes similarly contradictory attitudes toward the Sierra Leonean state in the postwar period, where routine criticisms of the state's inadequacy coexisted with the widespread belief in its indispensability.

3. HOME TRUTHS

1. Brown and Sáez, "Ebola Separations," explore different dimensions of separation and distancing during the West African Ebola epidemic, particularly in medical settings.

2. Farmer, "Ebola, the Spanish Flu, and the Memory of Disease," describes Ebola as the "caregivers disease."

3. The feeling of being stuck is widely ascribed as the central subjective experience of the crisis of youth in a variety of settings in Africa. See Hansen, "Getting Stuck in the Compound"; Mains, "Neoliberal Times"; and Sommers, *Stuck*.

4. Castro and Farmer, "Understanding and Addressing AIDS-Related Stigma," critique the popularization of the concept of stigmatization in public health discourse, pointing out the ways that it can mask deeper and more complex social inequalities.

5. The home is highly underrepresented in the study of contemporary male youths in urban Africa. Recent work has begun to acknowledge the significance and complexities of this space in economic, social, and cultural terms. See Masquelier, *Fada*; and Smith, *To Be a Man Is Not a One-Day Job*.

6. Anthropological scholarship has emphasized the ways that ambiguity in domestic settings in a range of different contexts is connected to wider, often violent, historical events and processes: the Atlantic slave trade in study of a Mende village in Sierra Leone by Ferme, *The Underneath of Things*; partition and the massacre of Sikhs in the study in India by Das, *Life and Words*; the forms of financialization associated with neoliberalism in the study of South Africa by James, *Money for Nothing*, and of urban Chile in the study by Han, *Life in Debt*; and political rupture and domestic dislocation in the study of rural China by Bruckermann, *Claiming Homes*.

7. As Jane Guyer, *Marginal Gains*, reveals, there is a long regional history of status recognition intersecting complexly with registers of exchange based on contradictory logics in Atlantic Africa. Marginal gains are secured through strategically positioning oneself at the interface of different registers of exchange.

8. For Geschiere, *Witchcraft, Intimacy, and Trust*, witchcraft in Africa, which is described as the "dark side of kinship," is a powerful modern discourse on the ways that relations of intimacy hold malevolent potential.

9. Turner, *Schism and Continuity in an African Society*, 93.

10. Cooper, "Sitting and Standing," argues that creative, often embodied, ways to "fix" the family in Africa are prevalent as a result of social, economic, and political upheavals.

4. EXTRAORDINARY ORDINARY

1. There is a growing literature on public authority and crisis in Africa, which emphasizes how multiple authorities oversee day-to-day governance in contexts were state capacity is limited. For an overview, see Kirk and Allen, "Public Authority in Africa." For a discussion of public authority during COVID-19 in Uganda, see Kirk et al., "Crisis Responses, Opportunity, and Public Authority during Covid-19's First Wave in Uganda, the Democratic Republic of Congo, and South Sudan."

2. On gender inequalities in global health governance and on the ground during the Ebola epidemic in West Africa, see Harman, "Ebola, Gender and Conspicuously Invisible Women in Global Health Governance," and Ibrahim, "'I Am a Woman. How Can I Not Help?'"

3. Shepler, "'We Know Who Is Eating the Ebola Money!," argues that Ebola money was a novel way of knowing the state in Sierra Leone during the epidemic.

4. On the difference between statistical and evaluative normal, see Warner, *The Trouble with Normal*.

5. Ferme, "The Violence of Numbers," 555–57.

6. Bolten. *I Did It to Save My Life*.

7. Bolten, "The Agricultural Impasse."

8. On social responses to conflict in different African contexts, see Lubkemann, *Culture in Chaos*; Porter, *After Rape*; and Vigh, "Crisis and Chronicity." In more general terms, Hage, "Waiting Out the Crisis," points to the value often ascribed to waiting out a crisis in the contemporary world.

9. For more on the complexities and challenges of pregnancy and childbirth during the Ebola emergency, see Black, *Belly Woman*; McKay et al., "Family Planning in the Sierra Leone Ebola Outbreak"; and Schwartz, Anoko, and Abramowitz, *Pregnant in the Time of Ebola*.

10. For analysis of how being educated as a source of status for young people in Uganda beyond the sphere of formal work resonates, see Jones, "Education as Identity."

11. For an ethnographic perspective on the everyday uncertainties facing ordinary Africans, see Cooper and Pratten, *Ethnographies of Uncertainties in Africa*.

12. Turner. *The Anthropology of Performance*, 42.

13. Guyer, "Prophecy and the Near Future."

14. This dovetails with the observation by Engelke, "Secular Shadows," that the "immanent" temporal orientation associated with secularism is underrepresented in Africanists debates, which have tended to center on religious temporalities.

15. Bornstein and Redfield, *Forces of Compassion*, identify the immediate future as the dominant temporality of humanitarian action.

5. BLACK AND WHITE DEATH

1. For more on the Bangura family compound, see chapter 2 in this volume.

2. Cohen, *The Politics of Elite Culture*, 68.

3. Anthropological analysis of good death, following the Durkheimian analysis of second burials in Hertz, *Death and the Right Hand*, has emphasized the close relationship between the performance of proper postdeath ritual and the maintenance and reproduction of social order. This is achieved by exerting ritual order in the face of abrupt and unpredictable biological death and, as Bloch and Parry, *Death and the Regeneration of Life*, explore, harnessing the regenerative powers of ritual to compensate for the loss of individuals by reinstalling them in the collective consciousness.

4. Sophocles's Antigone is a prime literary illustration of the risks of bad death, when the protagonist attempts to illegally perform an honorable burial for her brother—the disgraced loser of Thebes's civil war—against the orders of her uncle, King Creon. The ensuing disorder is characterized as a disease, tragically wiping out Creon's family and threatening social order at large: "the entire city is gripped by a violent disease" (*Antigone* II.114).

5. Fairhead, "Understanding Social Resistance to the Ebola Response in the Forest Region of the Republic of Guinea."

6. Parker et al., "Ebola and Public Authority."

7. For more on cosmologies and practices around death in Sierra Leone, see Jackson, "The Identity of the Dead"; Little, *The Mende of Sierra Leone*; MacCormack, "Dying as Transformation to Ancestorhood"; Richards, "A Matter of Grave Concern?"; and Spencer, "Invisible Enemy."

8. At our first encounter, I was surprised to discover that the German was Black, and he was surprised to discover that the family's lodger was White. After some time in the neighborhood, I earned the somewhat lighthearted nickname "black man in the white man's skin," which spoke to prevalent nonessentialized understandings of race.

9. See the examination of challenges in reconciling mass death with traditional categories of death and practices of memorization in postwar Vietnam in Kwon, *After the Massacre*.

10. Studies of modern funerary practices in Africa have similarly highlighted the coexistence of contestation and negotiation between competing social and religious groups and authorities. See, for example, Jindra and Noret, *Funerals in Africa*; De Boeck, "Death Matters"; Pendle, *Spiritual Contestations*; Posel and Gupta, "The Life of the Corpse"; Smith, "Burials and Belonging in Nigeria"; and de Witte, *Long Live the Dead!*

11. Fanon, *Black Skin, White Masks*.

12. See ethnographies by Diggins, *Coastal Sierra Leone*; Ferme, *The Underneath of Things*; and Shaw, *Memories of the Slave Trade*.

13. Fassin, "Racialization."

14. On the embodied and material dimensions of burial and funerary ritual, see Engelke, "The Coffin Question"; Engelke, "The Anthropology of Death Revisited"; and Hallam, Hockey, and Howarth, *Beyond the Body*.

15. Gomez-Temesio, "Outliving Death," observed a similar resurgence of imagery associated with the slave trade, in particular the figure of the zombie, in Ebola treatment centers in Guinea.

16. Harris, *Sierra Leone*, 13.

17. Benton, "Risky Business," argues that humanitarianism in Sierra Leone reinforces racialized nonequivalence in the valuations of human life, which Hirsch, "Race and the Spatialisation of Risk during the 2013–2016 West African Ebola Epidemic," documents in the international response to Ebola. In a connected way, Ferme and Hoffman, "Hunter Militias and the International Human Rights Discourse in Sierra Leone and Beyond," observed how that human rights discourses after the civil war became locally meaningful in Sierra Leone in ways antithetical to the international organizations that promote the discourse, while Shaw, *Memories of the Slave Trade*, observed the resurgence of local ritual knowledge over Western education in the context of economic failings.

18. Enria, "The Ebola Crisis in Sierra Leone," identified internal contradictions between humanitarianism's dual agendas of securitization and community engagement during the Ebola emergency. On inequalities between local and international actors during the crisis, see Abdullah and Rashid, *Understanding West Africa's Ebola Epidemic*; Abramowitz, "Epidemics (Especially Ebola)"; Fairhead, "Understanding Social Resistance to the Ebola Response in the Forest Region of the Republic of Guinea"; and Richards, "A Matter of Grave Concern?"

6. ANTHROPOLOGY IN CRISIS

1. Erikson, "Cell Phones ≠ Self and Other Problems with Big Data Detection and Containment during Epidemics," identifies significant limitations in big data approaches to disease management in Sierra Leone.

2. See the overview of anthropological engagement on Ebola by Abramowitz, "Epidemics (Especially Ebola)," as well as the account and critique of the discipline's search for relevance by Benton, "Ebola at a Distance."

3. On militant anthropology, see, for example, Scheper-Hughes, "The Primacy of the Ethical." On anarchist anthropology, see Graeber, *Fragments on an Anarchist Anthropology*. On decolonial ethnography, see Bejarano et al., *Decolonizing Ethnography*.

4. On sexual violence and ethnographic research, see Schneider, "Sexual Violence during Research," based on her own fieldwork in Freetown. On a decolonial queer of color reflection on fieldwork, see Adjepong, "Invading Ethnography." On blackness and fieldwork in New York City, see Jackson, *Real Black*.

5. Ferguson, "Anthropology and Its Evil Twin?"

6. Jobson, "The Case for Letting Anthropology Burn."

7. Kovats-Bernat, "Negotiating Dangerous Fields."

8. Rabinow, *Reflections on Fieldwork in Morocco*, 166.

9. On improvisation in jazz music as a metaphor for doing ethnography, see Humphreys, Brown, and Hatch, "Is Ethnography Jazz?"

10. Evens and Handelman, *The Manchester School*.

11. Kapferer, "Situations, Crisis, and Anthropology of the Concrete," 122.

12. On challenges of doing research during the Ebola epidemic, see Bolten and Shepler, "Producing Ebola" and Martineau, Wilkinson, and Parker, "Epistemologies of Ebola." On the possibilities of doing research during emergencies, see Hoffman and Lubkemann, "Introduction: West-African Warscapes."

13. Pigg, "On Sitting and Doing."

14. Bear et al., *A Right to Care*.

15. Schneider, *A Critique of the Study of Kinship*.

16. Kuper, "We Need to Talk about Kinship."

17. Kleinman, *Rethinking Psychiatry: from Cultural Category to Personal Experience*.

CONCLUSION

1. Seligman et al., *Ritual and Its Consequences*.

Bibliography

Abbink, Jon, and Ineke van Kessel, eds. *Vanguard or Vandals: Youth, Politics, and Conflict in Africa*. Leiden: Brill, 2005.

Abdullah, Ibrahim, and Ismail Rashid, eds. *Understanding West Africa's Ebola Epidemic: Towards a Political Economy*. London: Zed Books, 2017.

Abramowitz, Sharon. "Epidemics (Especially Ebola)." *Annual Review of Anthropology* 46, no. 1 (2017): 421–55. https://doi.org/10.1146/annurev-anthro-102116-041616.

Adjepong, Anima. "Invading Ethnography: A Queer of Color Reflexive Practice." *Ethnography* 20, no. 1 (2019): 27–46. https://doi.org/10.1177/1466138117741502.

Agamben, Giorgio. *State of Exception*. Chicago: University of Chicago Press, 2005.

Allen, Tim. *Trial Justice: The International Criminal Court and the Lord's Resistance Army*. London: Zed Books, 2006.

Asiama, Seth Opuni. "Land Accessibility and Urban Agriculture in Freetown, Sierra Leone." *Journal of Science and Technology* 25, no. 2 (2006): 103–9. https://doi.org/10.4314/just.v25i2.32945.

Banton, Michael. *West African City: A Study of Tribal Life in Freetown*. London: Oxford University Press, 1957.

Bear, Laura, Deborah James, Nikita Simpson, Eileen Alexander, Jaskiran K. Bhogal, Rebecca E. Bowers, Fenella Cannell, Anishka Gheewala Lohiya, Insa Koch, Megan Laws, Johannes F. Lenhard, Nicholas J. Long, Alice Pearson, Farhan Samanani, Olivia Vicol, Jordan Vieira, Connor Watt, Milena Wuerth, Catherine Whittle, and Teodor Zidaru Bărbulescu. *A Right to Care: The Social Foundations of Recovery from Covid-19*. London: LSE Monograph, 2020.

Bejarano, Carolina Alonso, Lucia López Juárez, Mirian A. Mijangos García, and Daniel M. Goldstein. *Decolonizing Ethnography: Undocumented Immigrants and New Directions in Social Science*. Durham, NC: Duke University Press, 2019.

Benton, Adia. "Ebola at a Distance: A Pathographic Account of Anthropology's Relevance." *Anthropological Quarterly* 90, no. 2 (2017): 495–524. https://doi.org/10.1353/anq.2017.0028.

Benton, Adia. *HIV Exceptionalism: Development through Disease in Sierra Leone*. Minneapolis: University of Minnesota Press, 2015.

Benton, Adia. "Risky Business: Race, Nonequivalence and the Humanitarian Politics of Life." *Visual Anthropology* 29, no. 2 (2016): 187–203. https://doi.org/10.1080/08949468.2016.1131523.

Benton, Adia. "Whose Security? Militarization and Securitization during West Africa's Ebola Outbreak." In *The Politics of Fear: Médecins Sans Frontières and the West African Ebola Epidemic*, edited by Michiel Hofman, and Sokhieng Au, 25–50. New York: Oxford Academic, 2017.

Berlant, Lauren. *Cruel Optimism*. Durham, NC: Duke University Press, 2011.

Bjarnesen, Jesper, and Mats Utas. "Introduction Urban Kinship: The Micro-Politics of Proximity and Relatedness in African Cities." *Africa* 88, no. S1 (2018): S1–S11. https://doi.org/10.1017/S0001972017001115.

Black, Benjamin Oren. *Belly Woman: Birth, Blood and Ebola; The Untold Story*. London: Neem Tree, 2022.

Bloch, Maurice, and Jonathan Parry, eds. *Death and the Regeneration of Life*. Cambridge: Cambridge University Press, 1982.

Bolt, Maxim. *Zimbabwe's Migrants and South Africa's Border Farms: The Roots of Impermanence*. Cambridge: Cambridge University Press, 2017.

Bolten, Catherine. "The Agricultural Impasse: Creating 'Normal' Post-War Development in Northern Sierra Leone." *Journal of Political Ecology* 16, no. 1 (2009): 70–86. https://doi.org/10.2458/v16i1.21692.

Bolten, Catherine. *I Did It to Save My Life: Love and Survival in Sierra Leone*. Berkeley: University of California Press, 2012.

Bolten, Catherine. *Serious Youth in Sierra Leone: An Ethnography of Performance and Global Connection*. Oxford: Oxford University Press, 2020.

Bolten, Catherine, and Susan Shepler. "Producing Ebola: Creating Knowledge in and about an Epidemic." *Anthropological Quarterly* 90, no. 2 (2017): 349–68. https://doi.org/10.1353/anq.2017.0022.

Bornstein, Erica, and Peter Redfield. *Forces of Compassion: Humanitarianism between Ethics and Politics*. Santa Fe, NM: School for Advanced Research Press, 2011.

Brown, Hannah, and Almudena M. Sáez. "Ebola Separations: Trust, Crisis, and 'Social Distancing' in West Africa." *Journal of the Royal Anthropological Institute*, 27, no. 1 (2021): 9–29. https://doi.org/10.1111/1467-9655.13426.

Bruckermann, Charlotte. *Claiming Homes: Confronting Domicide in Rural China*. New York: Berghahn, 2019.

Bürge, Michael. "Riding the Narrow Tracks of Moral Life: Commercial Motorbike Riders in Makeni, Sierra Leone." *Africa Today* 58, no. 2 (2011): 58–95. https://doi.org/10.1353/at.2011.0049.

Calhoun, Craig. "The Idea of Emergency: Humanitarian Action and Global (Dis)Order." In *Contemporary States of Emergency: The Politics of Military and Humanitarian Interventions*, edited by Didier Fassin and Mariella Pandolfi, 29–58. New York: Zone Books, 2013.

Castro, Arachu, and Paul Farmer. "Understanding and Addressing AIDS-Related Stigma: From Anthropological Theory to Clinical Practice in Haiti." *American Journal of Public Health* 95, no. 1 (2005): 53–59. http://www.ncbi.nlm.nih.gov/pmc/articles/PMC1449851/.

Chigudu, Simukai. *The Political Life of an Epidemic: Cholera, Crisis and Citizenship in Zimbabwe*. Cambridge: Cambridge University Press, 2020.

Cohen, Abner. *The Politics of Elite Culture: Explorations in the Dramaturgy of Power in a Modern African Society*. Berkeley: University of California Press, 1981.

Comaroff, Jean, and John Comaroff. *Of Revelation and Revolution*. Chicago: University of Chicago Press, 1997.

Cooper, Elizabeth. "Sitting and Standing: How Families Are Fixing Trust in Uncertain Times." *Africa* 82, no. 3 (2012): 437–56. https://doi.org/10.1017/s0001972012000320.

Cooper, Elizabeth, and David Pratten, eds. *Ethnographies of Uncertainty in Africa*. Basingstoke, UK: Palgrave Macmillan, 2015.

Das, Veena. *Life and Words: Violence and the Descent into the Ordinary*. Berkeley: University of California Press, 2006.

De Boeck, Filip. "Death Matters: Intimacy, Violence and the Production of Social Knowledge by Urban Youth in the Democratic Republic of Congo." In *Can There Be Life without Others?*, edited by António P. Ribeiro, 44–64. Manchester, UK: Carcanet, 2009.

De Boeck, Filip, and Marie-Francoise Plissart. *Kinshasa*. Ghent: Ludion, 2006.

de Witte, Marleen. *Long Live the Dead! Changing Funeral Celebrations in Asante (Ghana)*. Amsterdam: Aksant Academic Publishers, 2001.

Diggins, Jennifer. *Coastal Sierra Leone: Materiality and the Unseen in Maritime West Africa*. Cambridge: Cambridge University Press, 2018.

Di Nunzio, Marco. *The Act of Living: Street Life, Marginality, and Development in Urban Ethiopia*. Ithaca, NY: Cornell University Press, 2019.

Durham, Deborah. "Disappearing Youth: Youth as a Social Shifter in Botswana." *American Ethnologist* 31, no. 4 (2004): 589–605. https://doi.org/10.1525/ae.2004.31.4.589.

Engelke, Matthew. "The Anthropology of Death Revisited." *Annual Review of Anthropology* 48, no. 1 (2019): 29–44. https://doi.org/10.1146/annurev-anthro-102218-011420.

Engelke, Matthew. "The Coffin Question: Death and Materiality in Humanist Funerals." *Material Religion* 11, no. 1 (2015): 26–28. https://doi.org/10.2752/205393215X14259900061553.

Engelke, Matthew. "Secular Shadows: African, Immanent, Post-Colonial." *Critical Research on Religion* 3, no. 1 (2015): 86–100. https://doi.org/10.1177/2050303215584229.

Englund, Harri. *Prisoners of Freedom: Human Rights and the African Poor*. Berkeley: University of California Press, 2006.

Enria, Luisa. "The Ebola Crisis in Sierra Leone: Mediating Containment and Engagement in Humanitarian Emergencies." *Development and Change* 50, no. 6 (2019): 1602–23. https://doi.org/10.1111/dech.12538.

Enria, Luisa. *The Politics of Work in a Post-Conflict State: Youth, Labour and Violence in Sierra Leone*. Woodbridge, UK: Boydell and Brewer, 2018.

Erikson, Susan L. "Cell Phones ≠ Self and Other Problems with Big Data Detection and Containment during Epidemics." *Medical Anthropology Quarterly* 32, no. 3 (2018): 315–39. https://doi.org/10.1111/maq.12440.

Erikson, Susan L. "Global Health Futures? Reckoning with a Pandemic Bond." *Medicine Anthropology Theory* 6 (2019). https://doi.org/10.17157/mat.6.3.664.

Evans-Pritchard, E. E. *The Nuer*. Oxford: Oxford University Press, 1940.

Evens, Terence M. S., and Don Handelman. *The Manchester School: Practice and Ethnographic Praxis in Anthropology*. New York: Berghahn Books, 2008.

Fairhead, James. "Understanding Social Resistance to the Ebola Response in the Forest Region of the Republic of Guinea: An Anthropological Perspective." *African Studies Review* 59, no. 2 (2016): 7–31. https://doi.org/10.1017/asr.2016.87.

Fanon, Frantz. *Black Skin, White Masks*. New York: Grove, 2019.

Farmer, Paul. "Ebola, the Spanish Flu, and the Memory of Disease." *Critical Inquiry* 46, no. 1 (2019): 56–70. https://doi.org/10.1086/705301.

Farmer, Paul. *Fevers, Feuds, and Diamonds: Ebola and the Ravages of History*. New York: Farrar, Straus and Giroux, 2020.

Farmer, Paul. *Infections and Inequalities: The Modern Plagues*. Berkeley: University of California Press, 1999.

Farmer, Paul, Arthur Kleinman, Jim Kim, and Matthew Basilico. *Reimagining Global Health: An Introduction*. Berkeley: University of California Press, 2013.

Fassin, Didier. "Racialization: How to Do Races with Bodies." In *A Companion to the Anthropology of the Body and Embodiment*, edited by Frances E. Mascia-Lees, 419–34. Chichester, West Sussex, UK: Wiley-Blackwell, 2011.

Fassin, Didier. *When Bodies Remember: Experiences and Politics of AIDS in South Africa*. Berkeley: University of California Press, 2007.

Ferguson, James. "Anthropology and Its Evil Twin? Development and the Constitution of an Institution." In *International Development and the Social Sciences: Essays on the History and Politics of Knowledge*, edited by Frederick Cooper and Randall Packard, 150–175. Berkeley: University of California Press, 1997.

Ferguson, James. *The Anti-Politics Machine: "Development," Depoliticization, and Bureaucratic Power in Lesotho*. Cambridge: Cambridge University Press, 1990.

Ferme, Mariane C. *Out of War: Violence, Trauma, and the Political Imagination in Sierra Leone*. Berkeley: University of California Press, 2018.

Ferme, Mariane C. *The Underneath of Things: Violence, History, and the Everyday in Sierra Leone*. Berkeley: University of California Press, 2001.

Ferme, Mariane C. "The Violence of Numbers: Consensus, Competition, and the Negotiation of Disputes in Sierra Leone." *Cahiers d'Études Africaines* 38, no. 150/152 (1998): 555–80. https://doi.org/10.3406/cea.1998.1814.

Ferme, Mariane C., and Danny Hoffman. "Hunter Militias and the International Human Rights Discourse in Sierra Leone and Beyond." *Africa Today* 50, no. 1 (2004): 73–95. https://doi.org/10.2979/AFT.2004.50.4.72.

Fortes, Meyer. *Kinship and the Social Order: The Legacy of Lewis Henry Morgan*. London: Routledge, 1969.

Fortes, Meyer. *The Web of Kinship among the Tallensi*. London: Oxford University Press, 1949.

Fyfe, Christopher. *A History of Sierra Leone*. Oxford: Oxford University Press, 1962.

Gardner, Katy. *Discordant Development: Global Capitalism and the Struggle for Connection in Bangladesh*. London: Pluto, 2012.

Gershon, Ilana. "Porous Social Orders." *American Ethnologist* 46, no. 4 (2019): 404–16. https://doi.org/10.1111/amet.12829.

Geschiere, Peter. *Witchcraft, Intimacy, and Trust*. Chicago: University of Chicago Press, 2013.

Gomez-Temesio, Veronica. "Outliving Death: Ebola, Zombies, and the Politics of Saving Lives." *American Anthropologist* 120, no. 4 (2018): 738–51. https://doi.org/10.1111/aman.13126.

Graeber, David. *Fragments of an Anarchist Anthropology*. Chicago: Prickly Paradigm, 2004.

Guyer, Jane I. *Marginal Gains: Monetary Transactions in Atlantic Africa*. Chicago: University of Chicago Press, 2004.

Guyer, Jane I. "Prophecy and the Near Future: Thoughts on Macroeconomic, Evangelical, and Punctuated Time." *American Ethnologist* 34, no.3 (2007): 409–21. https://doi.org/10.1525/ae.2007.34.3.409.

Hage, Ghassan. "Waiting Out the Crisis: On Stuckedness and Governmentality." In *Waiting*, edited by Ghassan Hage, 97–106. Melbourne: Melbourne University Press, 2009.

Hallam, Elizabeth, Jenny Hockey, and Glennys Howarth. *Beyond the Body: Death and Social Identity*. London: Routledge, 1999.

Han, Clara. *Life in Debt: Times of Care and Violence in Neoliberal Chile*. Berkeley: University of California Press, 2012.

Hansen, Karen Tranberg. "Getting Stuck in the Compound: Some Odds against Social Adulthood in Lusaka, Zambia." *Africa Today* 51, no. 4 (2005): 3–16. https://doi.org/10.1353/at.2005.0039.

Harman, Sophie. "Ebola, Gender and Conspicuously Invisible Women in Global Health Governance." *Third World Quarterly* 37, no. 3 (2016): 524–41. https://doi.org/10.1080/01436597.2015.1108827.

Harris, David. *Sierra Leone: A Political History*. London: C. Hurst, 2013.

Hertz, Robert. *Death and the Right Hand*. London: Cohen and West, [1909] 1960.

Hirsch, Lioba A. "Race and the Spatialisation of Risk during the 2013–2016 West African Ebola Epidemic." *Health & Place* 67 (2021): 102499. https://doi.org/10.1016/j.healthplace.2020.102499.

Hoffman, Danny. *The War Machines: Young Men and Violence in Sierra Leone and Liberia*. Durham, NC: Duke University Press, 2011.

Hoffman, Danny, and Stephen Lubkemann. "Introduction: West-African Warscapes: Warscape Ethnography in West Africa and the Anthropology of 'Events.'" *Anthropological Quarterly* 78, no. 2 (2005): 315–27. https://doi.org/10.1353/anq.2005.0024.

Honwana, Alcinda. *Youth, Waithood and Protest Movements in Africa*. London: International African Institute, 2013.

Honwana, Alcinda, and Filip De Boeck, eds. *Makers and Breakers: Children and Youth in Postcolonial Africa*. Oxford: James Currey, 2005.

Hopkins, Donald R., Donald J. Millar, Michael J. Lane, and Evelyn C. Cummings. "Smallpox in Sierra Leone." *American Journal of Tropical Medicine and Hygiene* 20, no. 5 (1971): 689–96. https://doi.org/10.4269/ajtmh.1971.20.689.

Humphreys, Michael, Andrew Brown, and Mary J. Hatch. "Is Ethnography Jazz?" *Organization* 10, no. 1 (2003): 5–31. https://doi.org/10.1177/1350508403010001369.

Hunter, Mark. *Love in the Time of Aids: Inequality, Gender, and Rights in South Africa*. Bloomington: Indiana University Press, 2010.

Ibrahim, Aisha Fofana. "'I Am a Woman. How Can I Not help?' Gender Performance and the Spread of Ebola in Sierra Leone." In *Understanding West Africa's Ebola Epidemic: Towards a Political Economy*, edited by Ibrahim Abdullah and Ismail Rashid, 163–86. London: Zed Books, 2017.

Jackson, John L. *Real Black: Adventures in Racial Sincerity*. Chicago: University of Chicago Press, 2005.

Jackson, Michael. "The Identity of the Dead: Aspects of Mortuary Ritual in a West African Society." *Cahiers d'Études Africaines* 17 (1977): 271–97. https://doi.org/10.3406/CEA.1977.2454.

Jackson, Michael. *Life within Limits: Well-being in a World of Want*. Durham, NC: Duke University Press, 2011.

James, Deborah. *Money from Nothing: Indebtedness and Aspiration in South Africa*. Stanford, CA: Stanford University Press, 2014.

James, Deborah. "The Return of the Broker: Consensus, Hierarchy, and Choice in South African Land Reform." *Journal of the Royal Anthropological Institute* 17, no. 1 (2011): 318–38. https://doi.org/10.1111/j.1467-9655.2011.01682.x.

James, Deborah. *Songs of the Women Migrants: Performance and Identity in South Africa*. Edinburgh, UK: Edinburgh University Pres, 1999.

Janson, Marloes. *Islam, Youth and Modernity in the Gambia: The Tablighi Jama'at*. Cambridge: Cambridge University Press, 2013.

Jindra, Michael, and Joël Noret. *Funerals in Africa: Explorations of a Social Phenomenon*. New York: Berghahn Books, 2011.

Jobson, Ryan C. "The Case for Letting Anthropology Burn: Sociocultural Anthropology in 2019." *American Anthropologist* 122, no. 2 (2020): 259–71. https://doi.org/10.1111/aman.13398.

Johnson-Hanks, Jennifer. "On the Limits of Life Stages in Ethnography: Toward a Theory of Vital Conjunctures." *American Anthropologist* 104, no. 3 (2002): 865–80. https://doi.org/10.1525/aa.2002.104.3.865.

Jones, Ben. "Education as Identity: The Scaffolding of 'Being Educated' in Eastern Uganda." *American Ethnologist* 50, no. 2 (2023): 285–96. https://doi.org/10.1111/amet.13151.

Kapesea, Robby, and Thomas McNamara. "'We Are Not Just a Union, We Are a Family': Class, Kinship and Tribe in Zambia's Mining Unions." *Dialectical Anthropology* 44 (2020):153–72. https://doi.org/10.1007/s10624-019-09578-x.

Kapferer, Bruce. "Situations, Crisis, and Anthropology of the Concrete: The Contribution of Max Gluckman." In *The Manchester School: Practice and Ethnographic Praxis in Anthropology*, edited by Terence. M. S. Evens and Don Handelman, 118–55. New York: Berghahn Books, 2008.

Kirk, Tom, and Tim Allen. "Public Authority in Africa." In *Routledge Handbook of Public Policy in Africa*, edited by Gedion Onyango, 57–67. New York: Routledge, 2022.

Kirk, Tom, Duncan Green, Tim Allen, Tatiana Carayannis, José Bazonzi, José Ndala, Patrycja Stys, et al. "Crisis Responses, Opportunity, and Public Authority during Covid-19's First Wave in Uganda, the Democratic Republic of Congo, and South Sudan." *Disasters* 45, no. S1 (2021). https://doi.org/10.1111/disa.12513.

Klein, Naomi. *The Shock Doctrine: The Rise of Disaster Capitalism*. New York: Metropolitan Books, 2007.

Kleinman, Arthur. *Rethinking Psychiatry: From Cultural Category to Personal Experience*. New York: Free Press, 1988.

Kovats-Bernat, J. Christopher. "Negotiating Dangerous Fields: Pragmatic Strategies for Fieldwork amid Violence and Terror." *American Anthropologist* 104, no. 1 (2002): 208–22. https://doi.org/10.1525/aa.2002.104.1.208.

Kuper, Adam. "We Need to Talk about Kinship." *Anthropology of This Century*, no. 23 (2018): http://aotcpress.com/articles/talk-kinship/.

Kwon, Heonik. *After the Massacre: Commemoration and Consolation in Ha My and My Lai*. Berkeley: University of California Press, 2006.

Lazar, Sian. 2018. "A 'Kinship Anthropology of Politics'? Interest, the Collective Self and Kinship in Argentine Unions." *Journal of the Royal Anthropology Institute* (*N.S.*) 24: 256–74. https://doi.org/10.1111/1467-9655.12809.

Leach, Melissa. *Rainforest Relations: Gender and Resource Use among the Mende of Gola, Sierra Leone*. Edinburgh, UK: Edinburgh University Press, 1994.

Little, Kenneth. *The Mende of Sierra Leone*. London: Routledge, 1967.

Lovejoy, Paul E., and Jan S. Hogendorn. *Slow Death for Slavery: The Course of Abolition in Northern Nigeria, 1897–1936*. Cambridge: Cambridge University Press, 2011.

Lubkemann, Stephen C. *Culture in Chaos: An Anthropology of the Social Condition in War*. Chicago: University of Chicago Press, 2007.

MacCormack, Carol. P. "Dying as Transformation to Ancestorhood: The Sherbro Coast of Sierra Leone." In *Sterben und Tod Eine kulturvergleichende Analyse*, edited by Dorothea Sich, 117–26. Wiesbaden: Springer Vieweg Verlag, 1986. https://doi.org/10.1007/978-3-322-88770-2_14.

Mains, Daniel. "Neoliberal Times: Progress, Boredom, and Shame among Young Men in Urban Ethiopia." *American Ethnologist* 34, no. 4 (2007): 659–73. https://doi.org/10.1525/ae.2007.34.4.659.

Marcis, Frédéric Le, Luisa Enria, Sharon Abramowitz, Almudena-Mari Saez, and Sylvain Landry B. Faye. "Three Acts of Resistance during the 2014–16 West Africa Ebola Epidemic." *Journal of Humanitarian Affairs* 1, no. 2 (2019): 23–31. https://doi.org/10.7227/jha.014.

Martineau, Frederick, Annie Wilkinson, and Melissa Parker. "Epistemologies of Ebola: Reflections on the Experience of the Ebola Response Anthropology Platform." *Anthropological Quarterly* 90, no. 1 (2017): 475–94. https://doi.org/10.1353/anq.2017.0027.

Masquelier, Adeline. *Fada: Boredom and Belonging in Niger*. Chicago: University of Chicago Press, 2019.

Mbembe, Achille, and Janet Roitman. "Figures of the Subject in Times of Crisis." *Public Culture* 7, no. 2 (1995): 323–52. https://doi.org/10.1215/08992363-7-2-323.

McKay, Gillian, Luisa Enria, Sara L. Nam, Maseray Fofanah, Suliaman Gbonnie Conteh, and Shelley Lees. "Family Planning in the Sierra Leone Ebola Outbreak: Women's Proximal and Distal Reasoning." *Studies in Family Planning* 53, no. 4 (2022): 575–93. https://doi.org/10.1111/sifp.12210.

Mead, Margaret. *Coming of Age in Samoa: A Psychological Study of Primitive Youth for Western Civilization*. New York: William Morrow, 1928.

Meillassoux, Claude. *Maidens, Meal and Money: Capitalism and the Domestic Economy.* Cambridge: Cambridge University Press, 1981.

Mieth, Friederike. "Bringing Justice and Enforcing Peace? An Ethnographic Perspective on the Impact of the Special Court for Sierra Leone." *International Journal of Conflict and Violence* 7, no. 1 (2013): 10–22. https://doi.org/https://doi.org/10.4119/ijcv-2946.

Menzel, Anne. "Between Ex-Combatization and Opportunities for Peace: The Double-Edged Qualities of Motorcycle-Taxi Driving in Urban Postwar Sierra Leone." *Africa Today* 58, no. 2 (2011): 96–127. https://doi.org/10.1353/at.2011.005.1.

Narotzky, Susana, and Niko Besnier. "Crisis, Value, and Hope: Rethinking the Economy; An Introduction to Supplement 9." *Current Anthropology* 55, no. S9 (2014): S4–16. https://doi.org/10.1086/676327.

Nuttall, Sarah, and Achille Mbembe. *Johannesburg.* Durham, NC: Duke University Press, 2008.

Parker, Melissa, Moses Baluku, Bono E. Ozunga, Bob Okello, Peter Kermundu, Grace Akello, Hayley MacGregor, Melissa Leach, and Tim Allen. "Epidemics and the Military: Responding to Covid-19 in Uganda." *Social Science & Medicine* 314 (2022): 115482. https://doi.org/10.1016/j.socscimed.2022.115482.

Parker, Melissa, Tommy Matthew Hanson, Ahmed Vandi, Lawrence Sao Babawo, and Tim Allen. "Ebola and Public Authority: Saving Loved Ones in Sierra Leone." *Medical Anthropology* 38, no. 5 (2019): 440–54. https://doi.org/10.1080/01459740.2019.1609472.

Pendle, Naomi R. *Spiritual Contestations: The Violence of Peace in South Sudan.* Oxford: James Currey, 2023.

Peters, Krijn. "From Weapons to Wheels: Young Sierra Leonean Ex-combatants Become Motorbike Taxi-Riders." *Journal of Peace, Conflict and Development* 10, no. 10 (2007): 1–23. https://edepot.wur.nl/26906.

Peters, Krijn. *War and the Crisis of Youth in Sierra Leone.* Cambridge: Cambridge University Press, 2011.

Pigg, Stacy L. "On Sitting and Doing: Ethnography as Action in Global Health." *Social Science and Medicine* 99, no. 1 (2013): 127–34. https://doi.org/10.1016/j.socscimed.2013.07.018.

Polman, Linda. *The Crisis Caravan: What's Wrong with Humanitarian Aid?* New York: Picador, 2011.

Porter, Holly. *After Rape: Violence, Justice, and Social Harmony in Uganda.* Cambridge: Cambridge University Press, 2016.

Posel, Deborah, and Pamila Gupta. "The Life of the Corpse: Framing Reflections and Questions." *African Studies* 68, no. 3 (2009): 299–309. https://doi.org/10.1080/00020180903381248.

Rabinow, Paul. *Reflections on Fieldwork in Morocco.* Berkeley: University of California Press, 1977.

Rashid, Ismail. "Epidemics and Resistance in Colonial Sierra Leone during the First World War." *Canadian Journal of African Studies* 45, no. 3 (2011): 415–39. https://doi.org/10.1080/00083968.2011.10541064.

Rashid, Ismail. "Patterns of Rural Protest: Chiefs, Slaves and Peasants in Northwestern Sierra Leone, 1896–1956." PhD diss., McGill University, 1998.

Reece, Koreen M. "'We Are Seeing Things': Recognition, Risk and Reproducing Kinship in Botswana's Time of AIDS." *Africa* 89, no. 1 (2019): 40–60. https://doi.org/10.1017/S0001972018000694.

Richards, Paul. *Ebola: How a People's Science Helped End an Epidemic.* London: Zed Books, 2016.

Richards, Paul. *Fighting for the Rain Forest: War, Youth and Resources in Sierra Leone.* Portsmouth, NH: Heinemann, 1996.

Richards, Paul. "A Matter of Grave Concern? Charles Jedrej's Work on Mende Sodalities, and the Ebola Crisis." *Critical African Studies* 8, no. 1 (2016): 80–91. https://doi.org/10.1080/21681392.2016.1099021.

Rodney, Walter. *A History of the Upper Guinea Coast, 1545–1800.* New York: Monthly Review Press, 1970.

Roitman, Janet. *Anti-Crisis.* Durham, NC: Duke University Press, 2014.

Scheper-Hughes, Nancy. "The Primacy of the Ethical: Propositions for a Militant Anthropology." *Current Anthropology* 36, no.3 (1995): 409–40. https://escholarship.org/uc/item/2xq430hc.

Schneider, David M. *A Critique of the Study of Kinship.* Ann Arbor: University of Michigan Press, 1984.

Schneider, Luisa T. "Sexual Violence during Research: How the Unpredictability of Fieldwork and the Right to Risk Collides with Academic Bureaucracy and Expectations." *Critique of Anthropology* 40, no. 2 (2020): 173–93. https://doi.org/10.1177/0308275X20917272.

Schwartz, David A., Julienne Ngoundoung Anoko, and Sharon Alane Abramowitz. *Pregnant in the Time of Ebola: Women and Their Children in the 2013–2015 West African Epidemic.* Cham, Switzerland: Springer, 2019.

Seisay, Alhassan Lans and Mohamed Koblo Kamara. *Sierra Leone 2015: Population and Housing Census; Thematic Report on Mortality,* Statistics Sierra Leone (2017). https://www.statistics.sl/images/StatisticsSL/Documents/Census/2015/sl_2015_phc_thematic_report_on_mortality.pdf.

Seligman, Adam, Robert P. Weller, Michael Puett, and Bennett Simon. *Ritual and Its Consequences: An Essay on the Limits of Sincerity.* New York: Oxford University Press, 2008.

Shaw, Rosalind. *Memories of the Slave Trade: Ritual and the Historical Imagination in Sierra Leone.* Chicago: University of Chicago Press, 2002.

Shepler, Susan. *Childhood Deployed: Remaking Child Soldiers in Sierra Leone.* New York: New York University Press, 2014.

Shepler, Susan. "'We Know Who Is Eating the Ebola Money!': Corruption, the State, and the Ebola Response." *Anthropological Quarterly* 90, no. 2 (2017): 451–73. https://doi.org/10.1353/anq.2017.0026.

Simone, Aboumaliq. *City Life from Jakarta to Dakar.* New York: Routledge, 2010.

Smith, Daniel Jordan. "Burials and Belonging in Nigeria: Rural-Urban Relations and Social Inequality in a Contemporary African Ritual." *American Anthropologist* 106, no. 3 (2004): 569–79. https://doi.org/10.1525/aa.2004.106.3.569.

Smith, Daniel Jordan. *To Be a Man Is Not a One-Day Job: Masculinity, Money, and Intimacy in Nigeria.* Chicago: University of Chicago Press, 2017.

Sommers, Marc. *Stuck: Rwandan Youth and the Struggle for Adulthood.* Athens: University of Georgia Press, 2012.

Spencer, Sylvanus N. "Invisible Enemy: Translating Ebola Prevention and Control Measures in Sierra Leone." Working Papers Series 13. Leipzig: Deutsch-Französich Gesellschaft, 2015.

Stilwell, Sean. *Slavery and Slaving in African History.* New Approaches to African History. Cambridge: Cambridge University Press, 2014.

Tapscott, Rebecca. *Arbitrary States: Social Control and Modern Authoritarianism in Museveni's Uganda.* Oxford: Oxford University Press, 2021.

Turner, Victor. *The Anthropology of Performance.* New York: PAJ Publications, 1987.

Turner, Victor. *The Forest of Symbols: Aspects of Ndembu Ritual.* Ithaca, NY: Cornell University Press, 1967.

Turner, Victor. *Schism and Continuity in an African Society.* Manchester, UK: Manchester University Press for Rhodes–Livingstone Institute, 1957.

United Nations, Department of Economic and Social Affairs, Population Division. *Population Facts: Youth Population Trends and Sustainable Development* no. 1 (2015). https://www.un.org/esa/socdev/documents/youth/fact-sheets/YouthPOP.pdf.

United Nations Development Programme. *Assessing the Socio-economic Impacts of Ebola Virus Disease in Guinea, Liberia and Sierra Leone: The Road to Recovery* (2014). https://www.undp.org/sites/g/files/zskgke326/files/migration/africa/EVD -Synthesis-Report-23Dec2014.pdf.

Vaughan, Megan. *Curing Their Ills: African Illness and Colonial Power.* Cambridge, UK: Polity, 1991.

Vigh, Henrik E. "Crisis and Chronicity: Anthropological Perspectives on Continuous Conflict and Decline." *Ethnos* 7, no. 1 (2008): 5–24. https://doi.org/10.1080/0014 1840801927509.

Vigh, Henrik E. "Social Death and Violent Life Chances." In *Navigating Youth, Generating Adulthood: Social Becoming in an African Context*, edited by Catrine Christiansen, Mats Utas, and Henrik E. Vigh, 31–60. Berkeley: University of California Press, 2006.

Wald, Priscilla. *Contagious: Cultures, Carriers, and the Outbreak Narrative.* Durham, NC: Duke University Press, 2008.

Walsh, Sinéad, and Oliver Johnhon. *Getting to Zero: A Doctor and a Diplomat on the Ebola Frontline.* London: ZED, 2018.

Warner, Michael. *The Trouble with Normal: Sex, Politics, and the Ethics of Queer Life.* New York: Free Press, 1999.

Wilkinson, Annie, and James Fairhead. "Comparison of Social Resistance to Ebola Response in Sierra Leone and Guinea Suggests Explanations Lie in Political Configurations Not Culture." *Critical Public Health* 27, no. 1 (2016): 14–27. https://doi .org/10.1080/09581596.2016.1252034.

World Health Organization. "Ebola Response Roadmap," August 28, 2014. https://www .who.int/publications/i/item/10665-131596. https://www.who.int/csr/resources /publications/ebola/response-roadmap/en/.

Index

Note: Page numbers in *italics* refer to illustrative matter.